Navigating the
Program Evaluation Process
for PETE & Kinesiology:
A Roadmap for Success

Terry A. Senne • Jacalyn L. Lund

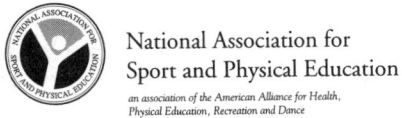

National Association for
Sport and Physical Education
*an association of the American Alliance for Health,
Physical Education, Recreation and Dance*

NASPE Sets the Standard

To order more copies of this book (stock # 304-10497):

Web: www.naspeinfo.org

E-mail: customerservice@aahperd.org

Phone: (800) 321-0789; (412) 741-1288 outside the United States

Fax: (412) 741-0609

Mail: AAHPERD Publications Fulfillment Center,
         P.O. Box 1020, Sewickley, PA 15143-1020

ISBN: 978-0-88314-954-6

Printed in the United States

Suggested citation for this book:

Senne, T.; Lund, J. (2012). *Navigating the program evaluation process for PETE & kinesiology: A roadmap for success.* Reston, VA.: National Association for Sport and Physical Education.

Dedication

This book is dedicated to our friend and mentor, De Raynes.

Contents

Preface

When most people think about program evaluation, they think about Commission on Accreditation of Allied Health Education Programs (CAAHEP) accreditation or the stressful on-site visit by the National Council for Accreditation of Teacher Education (NCATE). In fact, many physical education teacher education (PETE) faculty members measure time until retirement by the number of National Association for Sport and Physical Education (NASPE) program reports they will need to write before they enter their golden years.

There are, however, other reasons for undergoing program evaluation. University climates are changing, and budgets are decreasing. Instead of being almost fully funded, institutions increasingly must rely on grants and other sources of revenue. Also, the funds allocated by state legislatures are coming with more and more strings attached. Much like public schools, universities are being held accountable for student learning. As such, they are starting to add requirements for program evaluation and documentation of candidate performance. Deans are using program evaluation and documentation of candidate performance to justify additional faculty positions. Consider this scenario: A department chair is trying to convince the dean that a program in the department needs a new faculty position. Program enrollment has increased by 225 percent over the past four years, with no increase in the number of faculty members. Classes have doubled in size, to accommodate enrollment increases, and most classes — including advanced classes taken just prior to the internship semester — have at least 70 students in them. The increased class size has affected faculty member time and has resulted in decreased grant writing, decreased research productivity and less publication. The dean promises to increase the number of faculty positions if the chair provides evidence of program quality. In this case, providing program evaluation data to demonstrate excellence is the key to resolving issues created by an inadequate number of faculty positions. What data will make the most compelling case for program excellence?

Conducting a program evaluation and writing an accreditation report (or a program report for national recognition) are similar in many ways, yet they also differ somewhat. Writing an accreditation report involves conducting a program evaluation while adhering to specific guidelines outlined by the accrediting agency. Some program faculty members consider the accreditation process to be a rigorous challenge and a tedious and demanding exercise that is required to attain or retain national recognition or accreditation. It's often high-stakes in nature, and is conducted under extreme pressure and within limited time constraints. Thus, one difference between program evaluation and writing an accreditation report is the voluntary nature of the former.

The second difference resides in the fact that programs seek accreditation only periodically. For instance, some accredited programs are reviewed only once every seven years. Subsequently, program faculty members can choose not to evaluate their program on a continuous basis. Doing so, however, puts programs at risk of becoming outdated and/or losing their accreditation status. If program faculty members choose this option, they could miss opportunities to improve program and candidate quality. They also run the risk of not having enough data when it's time to begin another cycle of writing the accreditation report.

Conversely, if program evaluation is ongoing, regardless of whether an accreditation report is due, program faculty members can monitor results carefully while making timely programmatic modifications or changes. Ongoing program evaluation allows faculty members to monitor the program's pulse continuously to improve program quality while remaining relevant and current.

One final important point: Continuous improvement, as a practice, must begin at the faculty level, where primary responsibility for coursework resides. Program faculty members must examine, analyze and interpret the quality of course delivery and candidate performance. Reflective examination, analysis and interpretation must occur at the conclusion of every semester for all program courses taught. In-depth course evaluation, in addition to overall program assessment and evaluation, ensures a two-pronged approach (top-down and bottom-up) to continuous program improvement and development.

Chapter 1 of this book provides an overview of the program evaluation process. The next three chapters contain suggestions about developing assessments (Chapter 2), establishing rubrics and developing criteria for assessments (Chapter 3) and using assessment data for program improvement (Chapter 4). Chapter 5 provides a description of how to "unpack" NASPE's National Standards for Initial PETE (NASPE, 2009), while Chapter 6 outlines the requirements specific to writing a program report for NASPE national recognition. Finally, in Chapter 7, we share our best suggestions about putting the final report together, whether for internal or external program evaluation. The book concludes with a section that describes the development of an internal curriculum review (redesign) report using the process described in this book, along with the decisions and the rationale for each step.

We would like to thank those professionals who reviewed the initial draft of this book and offered many helpful suggestions to improve its quality. We appreciate their insight and feel that their ideas strengthened our original thoughts.

Now, in the spirit of continuous program development, we offer this book to assist program faculty members in the process. We have implemented all of the steps successfully at our own institutions and wish to share our ideas and suggestions to help you begin your journey of continuous program evaluation.

Let the journey begin!

Chapter 1
Orientation to Program Evaluation

Education at the university level is changing. Many of the changes result from increased emphasis on outcomes-based learning, in which real learning is measured instead of "seat time," or how many hours candidates attend any particular course. The journey begins here, with an overview of program evaluation.

Why program evaluation? Oden (2009) provides in eloquent Socratic fashion the rationale for why program faculty members should choose to go through the program evaluation or accreditation process:

> We are a collection of teachers and scholars seeking always to expand the boundaries of what counts as knowledge, promoting our students' learning and learning from them. So, why would we not wish to learn all we can about ourselves? What possible objection might we formulate to a process that allows us to discover our strengths and weaknesses, our successes and challenges, our wont constantly to change to meet a changing world? About the only thing we can predict about the future is that the future is unpredictable, so why not work together to shape an education that will prepare our students for such a future? (p. 38)

In this chapter, we provide an orientation to program evaluation and an overview of the process. The concept of program evaluation as a continuous cycle serves as the underlying theme. Specifically, we:

- Define program evaluation and its purposes.
- Clarify terms and definitions that we use throughout the book.
- Outline an eight-step program-evaluation process.
- Provide a strong rationale for implementing program evaluation as a continuous cycle.

Terms & Definitions

Throughout this book, we use a couple of sets of terms on a consistent basis. It makes sense to clarify and define them here. The first term that we use is "candidate." Defined, this refers to any college/university student enrolled in a degree program, whether it's teacher education, exercise science or any other degree program at the college/university level. We choose to use the term "candidate" instead of "student" to avoid confusion with a child or adolescent in the K-12 environment. We use the term "student" only in reference to K-12.

Likewise, we need to clarify the terms "accreditation" and "national recognition." We use the term "accreditation" when referring to an entity or agency that has the authority to determine which college/university programs qualify for accreditation, such as the Commission on Sport Management Accreditation (COSMA), or when referring to a teacher education unit that receives accreditation through NCATE. We use the term "national recognition" only in the context of addressing Specialized Professional Association (SPA) programs, such as NASPE's. SPAs may grant *national recognition* to college/university professional education programs that meet their standards.

Program Evaluation as a Continuous Cycle

In this book, we look broadly at program evaluation, viewing it as a process by which program faculty members can attain and maintain program improvement and quality. One can view program evaluation as a continuous process that does not end. It:

- Poses critical questions about academic program and candidate quality.
- Assesses specific program traits or characteristics (typically, based on standards).
- Gathers assessment data over time.
- Analyzes and interprets data.
- Helps program faculty render judgments about program quality.
- Helps program faculty make judgments regarding program and curricular changes that will improve the quality of the program and its candidates.
- Generates a cycle of continuous improvement.

What Is Program Evaluation?

Mizikaci (2006) defines program evaluation as:

> … a systematic operation of varying complexity involving data collection, observations and analyses, and culminating in a value judgment with regard to the quality of the program being evaluated, considered in its entirety, or through one or more of its components. (p. 41)

Program evaluation provides the means by which faculty members can render a judgment about the *quality* of their program and candidates. Initially, conducting a program evaluation provides academic programs with objective baseline data about program and candidate performance. Subsequently, based on identified strengths and weaknesses specific to national standards, state standards, or programmatic goals, faculty members can make necessary modifications and changes.

Purposes of Program Evaluation

Program evaluation can serve a variety of functions. It can:

- Examine a single programmatic aspect and, subsequently, use that information to make curricular decisions specific to the targeted aspect.
- Document evidence of institutional effectiveness (IE) for the department as part of the university's IE plan.
- Provide data beneficial to the departmental/unit yearly review.
- Produce data beneficial to the program itself, including data that:
  - Make a case for the program's viability by supplying substantive, objective data that offer support for maintaining it.
  - Justify the need for additional program support and/or resources.
- Provide data as part of program report documentation for national recognition through the SPA.
- Provide data and substantive program information for program, unit and/or institutional accreditation purposes, including that from NCATE, Southern Association of Colleges and Schools (SACS), American College of Sports Medicine (ACSM) and COSMA.
- Serve as a mechanism for prompting policy change.

The Program Evaluation Process

We offer the following eight-step process as a guide to program evaluation. These steps are generic in nature and apply across disciplines and academic programs. They are illustrated in Figure 1.1.

Step 1: Pose critical questions about program and candidate quality. Faculty members must determine thoughtfully what they want to know about the program and its candidates. What questions do they want addressed through this process? If faculty members define their purpose(s) clearly by asking explicit and accurate questions, the data are more likely to reveal accurate answers to the questions posed.

Figure 1.1. The Program Evaluation Process

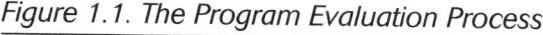

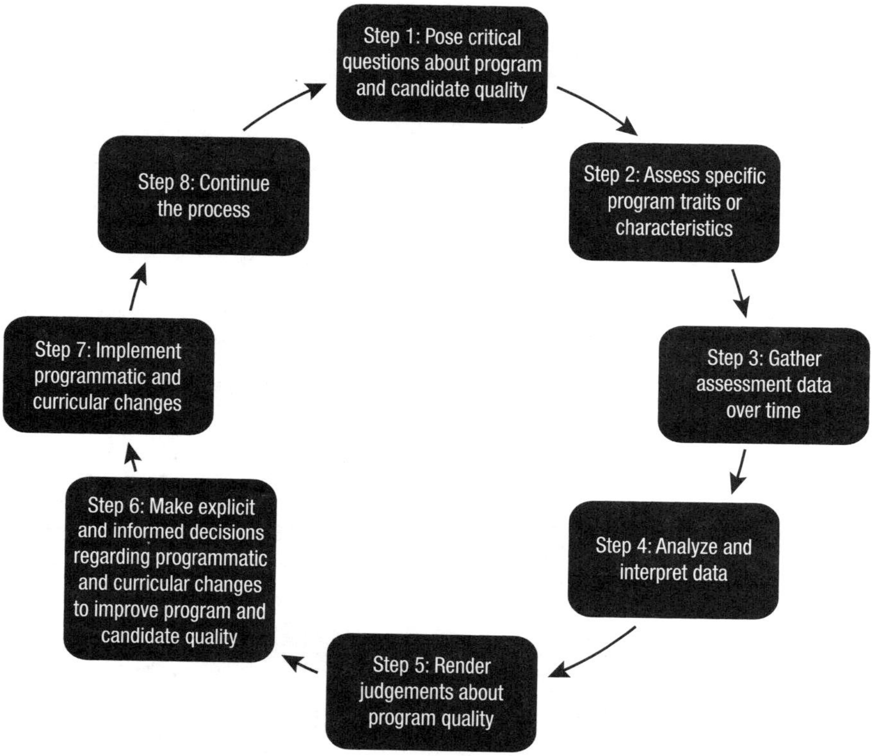

Step 2: Assess specific program traits or characteristics. As part of the program evaluation process, faculty members select traits or characteristics that align with the questions generated during Step 1. If seeking to improve program and candidate quality, faculty members should determine traits or characteristics of what the "end products" (graduates) should look like as candidates complete the degree program. They then use these traits or characteristics, in part, to select or develop program assessments that provide evidence specific to the selected traits/characteristics.

Often, for accreditation purposes, the questions are predetermined, and program faculty members are expected to show how well their candidates perform against a specific set of standards. Consequently, in this case, the question is "Do program candidates demonstrate an appropriate level of competency specific to the designated standards?"

This is a critical step in the program evaluation process. Selecting program traits or characteristics that don't align clearly with the intent of the program evaluation can produce evidence (data) that fails to provide an accurate picture of the program based on the questions posed. Regardless of the reason for conducting the program evaluation, it's essential that the program assessments used align directly with the standards, characteristics or traits guiding the program evaluation process, providing accurate data-driven information.

Step 3: Gather assessment data over time. Based on the program traits/characteristics identified and program assessments selected during Step 2, program faculty members collect data on the selected assessments over time. Looking at the data over time allows faculty members to determine whether any trends are occurring. Gathering data for only a single semester on a particular assessment, trait or characteristic doesn't provide faculty members with a clear sense of how the program is performing. In contrast, analyzing data from specific program assessments over several semesters helps to identify program and candidate strengths, as well as deficiencies. Only by providing a series of "snapshots" of selected program assessments over time does the big picture of program effectiveness become focused.

Step 4: Analyze and interpret data. What do the data reveal about the program and the quality of its candidates? Where are the program's strengths? What are its deficiencies or challenges? Are some curricular areas not being addressed?

Those are but a few of the questions that program faculty members must consider during Step 4 of the program evaluation process. They must conduct the analysis and interpretation component with great care, focusing on what fixes are necessary to make the program better, while also maintaining program strengths. Step 4 is crucial in the program evaluation process, because it's within this step that program faculty respond (based on data) to the questions posed in Step 1.

Step 5: Render judgments about program quality. This step is tied closely to Steps 4 and 6. Once data are analyzed and interpreted, program faculty members make a judgment about the program's quality. Valid and reliable data are essential to determining program quality. Step 5 requires faculty members to interpret the data correctly. Looking at data objectively is difficult, especially for those who are integral to the program's delivery, but if program faculty members allow biases to influence their judgments about program quality, the entire program evaluation process is for naught. Step 5, then, becomes the catalyst for Step 6.

Step 6: Make explicit and informed decisions regarding program and curricular changes to improve program and candidate quality. These decisions will vary by program and context. Deliberate initiatives taken in Step 6 will remediate any real or potential deficiencies and improve the program's quality. Sometimes, the decisions are curricular in nature; at other times, a decision might call for additional resources or an additional faculty member. In some cases, decisions can initiate changes in course sequencing. Typically, these decisions are program-specific. Making informed program and curricular decisions based on data instead of on fragmented anecdotal observations provides a strong objective platform for the resulting initiatives.

Step 7: Implement program and curricular changes. Once program faculty members have made the program and curricular decisions in Step 6, they implement the changes. Developing a timeline for implementation will help facilitate the process. Some changes are relatively easy and don't require action from the unit or university. Changes that necessitate catalog revisions and those that affect other content areas will take more time and effort to implement.

Step 8: Continue the process. Step 8 is the most important aspect of continuous program evaluation. Data collection and program improvement don't end once program and curricular changes are made to an academic program. Rather, program faculty members begin, once again, to pose questions about the changes made or to pose questions of a different nature, gather assessment data to respond to the questions, analyze and interpret data, render judgments, make additional decisions and implement changes. Thereby, they continue the evaluation process for continuous improvement.

Rationale for Continuous Program Development and Evaluation

Assessing the effectiveness and quality of an academic program through a systematic, data-driven approach of continuous program evaluation allows academic programs to stay current in discipline-specific content knowledge and its application, based on research and education-reform initiatives or state/federal mandates. Today's education climate demands that schools and institutions of higher education work diligently to address the needs of a changing society. Jewett, Bain and Ennis (1995) state that curricula should not be static; rather, they ought to be under revision constantly.

Continuous program evaluation, in addition to participation in the accreditation process, conveys the notion of a program changing when necessary to reflect the needs of society and the discipline. If, for example, program candidate performance starts to diminish relative to a specific standard or program goal, faculty members can see the trend immediately and respond by making timely curricular changes, instead of revisiting data only once every several years during the accreditation process.

Further, conducting program evaluation on a continuous basis allows program faculty members to take a systematic and holistic view of the total program. Most institutions have multiple faculty members teaching the various courses required for a program of study. Although individual faculty members have a good sense of what is happening in their own courses, they really don't have much of a sense of how candidates are performing in other degree-program courses. That can be particularly problematic for academic programs in which students must take some courses outside the department or school/college. Likewise, when a new faculty member joins a program, the content and the delivery of a course might change. Sometimes, changes are for the better; but, from time to time, candidate performance actually might decline. Participating in continuous program evaluation allows program faculty members to:

- Keep closer tabs on the various courses that contribute to the standards- or program-designated goals/criteria.
- Monitor candidate performance specific to the standards or program goals.
- Reflect on evidence (data) gathered.
- Make informed decisions about program changes to improve the quality of the program and its candidates.

Conclusion

Program evaluation can serve many purposes. Program faculty members can address multiple purposes concurrently (e.g., yearly program review, IE data, accreditation, support for additional resources/faculty) by implementing the eight-step approach to program evaluation. Continuous program evaluation provides a systematic, data-driven approach to improving program quality and candidate competency.

Chapter 2
Developing Measurable Program Outcomes

In the current education climate, it's important for academic programs to have stated outcomes and guidelines, regardless of whether they pursue accreditation or national recognition from external agencies. Many universities require programs to document student learning, and setting clear program goals is an important first step in that process.

Some accrediting agencies have developed standards designed to provide those guidelines and, thus, ensure consistency across universities and colleges offering similar degrees. For example, NASPE developed national standards for PETE programs. Similarly, accrediting bodies for other health-related programs, such as ACSM's Commission on Accreditation of Allied Health Education Programs (CAAHEP), developed standards describing the competencies for program graduates in their respective content areas (e.g., exercise science, athletic training). In contrast, while COSMA leaves the specifics of candidate competency up to each program, it does identify several content areas in which program graduates should demonstrate competence.

Along with having clearly articulated standards and outcomes, programs also must develop assessments and the criteria used to establish the level of excellence (often referred to as "rubrics" or "scoring guides") expected of candidates so that program faculty members know whether candidates are attaining desired levels of learning. Weak or inferior assessments tell little about program quality, and that often spells doom when the program tries to earn accreditation. In this chapter, we explain how to select or develop outcomes and the types of assessments that will allow program faculty members to measure program quality.

As we stated in Chapter 1, the purpose of this book is not just to help program faculty members develop an accreditation report, but rather to help them develop a sound curriculum designed to produce candidates who will succeed once they begin their careers. The seven-step process outlined in this chapter is designed to:

- Help program faculty members look critically at the needs of program graduates.
- Identify existing program content.
- Determine how program content aligns with the standards and/or program goals.
- Make necessary adjustments to existing content and courses to achieve the desired outcomes.

Seven Steps of Cirriculum Design

Step 1: Examine the needs of program completers. A good program stands for something. Program faculty members must ask: "What are we preparing candidates to do upon graduation?" For example, preparing candidates for the workplace requires different skills and coursework than preparing candidates for graduate study. Undergraduate programs in exercise science and sport administration might consist of more general goals than those of graduate programs, because they prepare candidates for a variety of careers in the profession.

For example, an undergraduate degree in exercise science can lead to a number of different specialty areas, including community-based fitness programs (e.g., YMCA, parks and recreation), corporate-based fitness and wellness programs (encompasses all types of businesses, from small businesses to major corporations), clinical programs (e.g., cardiac and pulmonary rehabilitation) and commercial fitness and wellness programs (e.g., Bally Total Fitness™, Gold's Gym™). Sport management programs also prepare candidates for a wide variety of jobs in the field, from selling tickets and planning promotional events to running programs at both the collegiate and professional sport levels.

Most candidates who earn an undergraduate degree in teacher education want to become teachers in a P-12 setting. Athletic training graduates also tend to have a narrow job focus: they want to rehabilitate clients. Identifying what the program prepares candidates to do upon graduation and then clarifying the needs of those graduates is a crucial first step in program evaluation.

Graduate programs in the fields named above generally include either a research component or training for specialized positions that require advanced skills. A discussion among program faculty members is an excellent way to clarify program intent and ensure that every faculty member is operating with the same set of assumptions.

- After faculty members determine what the program stands for, they need to develop a mission statement: a succinct statement that describes the program's purpose. Here are some examples:
- The Exercise Science Program seeks to prepare candidates for careers in corporate fitness, adult fitness, personal training, cardiac rehabilitation and related fields.
- The Health and Physical Education Program is designed to prepare candidates to

teach physical education in P-12 schools by offering high-quality education experiences and the opportunity to use skills and knowledge in a series of field experiences in diverse school contexts.

- The Athletic Training Program prepares students for career opportunities in the field of athletic training through coursework and laboratory experiences in preventing, managing, evaluating and rehabilitating athletic injuries.
- The Sport Management Program prepares graduates through rigorous coursework and internship experiences to enter the world of sport business in the professional or collegiate sport venue.

Writing a mission statement requires program faculty members to identify what they want program graduates to be able to do upon completing the program. The mission statement communicates the program's purpose to candidates, employers and others.

Step 2: Identify the essential content. The second step in the process of developing a high-quality course of study is to identify the knowledge, skills and dispositions that candidates should demonstrate. Those essential skills usually are identified using broad statements about content, which often are referred to as "content standards." As stated earlier, most content areas have established standards, certification or licensure requirements. A good program should align with these content standards to ensure that it includes the subject matter necessary for a comprehensive program of high quality. In addition to looking at those standards, program faculty members should take a hard look at what practitioners or researchers in the field are expected to do and then use that information to determine what content knowledge, skills and dispositions the program should address. They then can develop checklists for ensuring comprehensive coverage.

Although all the programs housed in kinesiology departments have standards or guidelines, each program has slightly different ways for addressing these.

- Teacher education programs must be accredited by the state (e.g., state department of education or equivalent) or a national agency (e.g., NCATE), using the standards specified. Typically, teacher education programs must expand the standards by unpacking them and their sub-standards or elements, using the process described in Chapter 5.
- In contrast, COSMA identifies content areas and leaves the development of content expectations to individual sport management programs.
- Exercise science programs that adhere to the ACSM guidelines must address specific knowledge, skills and abilities that have little, if any, need for unpacking or further explanation.
- Athletic trainers follow guidelines from the Commission on Accreditation of Athletic Training Education (CAATE) and, thus, also have little need to unpack standards.

When identifying the knowledge, skills and dispositions that a candidate should demonstrate, teacher education programs typically address three types of content knowledge. **Cognitive content knowledge** refers to basic knowledge of the science courses (e.g., anatomy, physiology, biomechanics, exercise physiology, motor development, motor learning), tactics of game play or knowledge needed to participate in other types of activity, knowledge of fitness, etc. Teacher candidates also must have the necessary **psychomotor skill knowledge** to participate in a variety of games from different categories (e.g., target, field, invasion, net/wall), dances, gymnastics and other types of physical activities (e.g., track and field, inline skating). Candidates also need the **pedagogical content knowledge** to teach a variety of games and activities to P-12 students.

Sport management program needs will depend on whether the program is preparing its candidates for working in the sports business, communications or media relations industries, or to work as athletic directors in a school district. Graduates often need skills associated with the world of business, such as marketing, finance, economics and accounting. Sport management candidates also benefit from coursework in facilities, facilities management, basic law and legal issues, and current topics in the field. Because the field is changing constantly, candidates need a broad base of coursework.

Exercise science candidates must have the knowledge, skills and abilities to pass a certification exam for the field. They also need a broad learning base because of the many diverse settings in which they can choose to work. Similarly, athletic training programs must prepare candidates to assess and rehabilitate injuries and teach rehab protocols to their clients. Both exercise science and athletic training graduates also often need course work in exercise psychology, which can help them work more effectively with their clients.

By identifying essential content knowledge that candidates will need, program faculty members can develop a systematic way of ensuring that graduates will have those skills and that knowledge. This content knowledge should align with the mission statement developed in Step 1.

Step 3: Identify courses to deliver the content knowledge. After identifying the essential content that graduates will need to succeed in their chosen careers, program faculty members must design the courses to deliver it. Most programs will see overlap in courses because several of the topics are universal to some content areas but are viewed from different perspectives. Also, a complex concept might be introduced in one course and then expanded on in a subsequent course. For example, if a PETE candidate learns about assessment in one course, subsequent methods courses should reinforce that learning as the candidate learns to implement the assessments and use the results to plan lessons. Exercise science students might learn what information electrocardiograms can provide in one class and then learn to administer and interpret the data in another. Content in athletic training, typically, is presented in a two-semester sequence, with candidates learning about a given content area in the first semester and using that knowledge in an applied/practicum setting the following semester.

To ensure that content knowledge is covered in a comprehensive and systematic manner, program faculty members should develop a matrix in which the alignment between the course and the content (developed in Step 2) is displayed visually. They also should develop a system for noting on the matrix when content is introduced in one course and reinforced in a subsequent course. Because of the interrelationship between content, program faculty members will want to indicate whether the course plays a major or minor role in contributing to the development of a given area of knowledge. Figure 2.1 provides an example of a partially developed matrix that shows both the courses a teacher candidate should take and the content that he/she should master.

Step 4: Examine the matrix to look for deficiencies, omissions or too much duplication. The matrix allows program faculty members to ascertain visually whether a topic has been addressed sufficiently. In some cases, faculty members might think that a topic is covered in depth in one class, while the matrix reveals only cursory coverage. The matrix can be useful in large programs, in which multiple instructors teach the same class. It also can show whether course content needs to be adjusted to ensure thorough coverage of a topic or content area.

In some instances, program faculty members might discover that faculty members thought someone else was addressing a topic when, in fact, no one was giving it the necessary amount of time. Sometimes, program faculty members can add missing content to existing courses. Sometimes, however, the deficiency might be so great that the need for an additional course becomes evident.

The matrix also can reveal redundancies: faculty members might realize that other courses address content areas covered in the courses they teach. Some redundancy provides a good review of important topics and program faculty members need to ensure that all topics have sufficient coverage. Using the matrix as the basis for discussing course content can provide faculty members the opportunity to determine whether they're covering program topics adequately and to ensure a balance between too much time and not enough time spent on a topic.

Step 5: Examine course objectives to ensure the delivery of content. To ensure that content knowledge is delivered in a course as specified by the matrix developed in Step 3, the course syllabus should feature an objective or outcome that states the intended learning relative to the content knowledge. Program faculty members should not assume that a particular course will address certain content knowledge or that candidates will have an adequate level of proficiency after taking the course. They should check the syllabus for each course to ensure that course objectives match the content area identified on the matrix. After performing an audit of course objectives using the matrix, faculty members will be able to determine where program objectives are being met and where they are not.

Within Step 5, program faculty members also should discuss the objectives currently used in various courses and determine whether to delete some of them. If an objective and/or assessment doesn't address a standard or element, or support a program goal, program faculty members should consider removing it from the syllabus.

Figure 2.1. Sample Matrix Showing Program Content & Courses

Course Number & Name	KH2130 Introductory course	KH2220 Anatomy	KH2230 Physiology	KH3010 Rhythms	
Class-Management Strategies					
Rules & routines					
Transitions					
Dealing with large classes				1	
Managing resources (time, space, equipment, activities, people)				2	
Dealing with inappropriate behavior	1			1	

1 = Topic is mentioned   2 = Topic is covered fully   3 = Application task for the topic or concept

Note: *This is only part of a much larger matrix intended to help assess all aspects of teacher education content and courses.*

Step 6: Examine course objectives to ensure that they are measurable. A good objective is a measurable objective. Mager (1984) suggests that a complete objective consists of three parts:

1. The performance. (What the student will be able to do.)
2. The situation. (The conditions under which the behavior is to occur.)
3. The criteria used to judge the performance.

All three must be present for an objective to be considered measurable.

Consider the following objectives that might be found in a program course:

1. Prior to teaching a lesson, the teacher candidate will have an understanding of the planning process.
2. The candidate will be able to take the blood pressure of a client.
3. The candidate will learn accounting principles needed for work in a sport business.

Although those objectives cover important topics, they're not measurable. They describe a performance but don't specify the conditions under which the performance is to take place or the level of competence expected. Consider these objectives:

1. Before beginning instruction, the teacher candidate will write a lesson plan using the department template (contextual overview, content development, assessments

KH3030 Team sports	KH3200 Beginning methods	KH3410 Assessment	KH4510 Elementary methods	KH4120 Secondary methods	KH4130 Health methods
	3		3	3	3
	2		3	3	3
	3		3	3	3
1	3	2	3	3	3
2	3		3	3	3

for the various learning tasks and reflections about the quality of the task) that meets the acceptable level of performance as stated in the lesson plan rubric.

2. Using approved techniques, the candidate will be able to assess blood pressure at both resting and exercising states within an accuracy of 10 mm of mercury.

3. The candidate will create a comprehensive budget feasibility study for adding a new sport to a college athletics department.

The second set of objectives is much more comprehensive and provides a clearer picture of intended course outcomes. The objectives are measurable so that program faculty members can determine whether candidates are acquiring the essential knowledge or skills that the course is supposed to deliver. Note the presence of an assessment in each objective to measure candidate learning. Developing measurable objectives is an important precursor to developing a sound program evaluation system. For the objectives to be measurable, they should state the level of performance desired.

The first objective addresses criteria for acceptable performance in a different way than do the other two objectives. The task is to write a lesson plan using the department template. Although the objective doesn't state the criteria for the assessment, it does state that the lesson plan will be evaluated using a set of external criteria (e.g., the rubric). The objective articulates one of the course's goals and specifies an assessment with an expected level of performance that provides a viable measure of learning.

Program faculty members also can use this technique for writing course objectives in other program areas. For example, the objective could describe performance during an internship and then reference the criteria that are found on a comprehensive rubric. The level of performance stated on the objective would be: "The intern will perform at the acceptable level of the rubric used to evaluate the experience." When an assessment uses complex criteria for evaluation, objectives can reference an external document to indicate the desired level of performance. Chapter 3 explains in detail how to develop rubrics, or scoring guides, for assessments.

Step 7: Identify assessments to measure whether graduates meet the desired outcomes. In this step, program faculty members should determine how they will ascertain whether candidates have met the acceptable level for the essential content that the program has identified. Generally, two sources are available for program evaluation data:

1. Assessments that use the knowledge from several courses but are not tied to a specific course.
2. Assessments that are connected to specific classes.

Assessments Not Tied to a Specific Course

The comprehensive certification exam (e.g., ACSM's certification exam) that some exercise science programs require of candidates is one example of an assessment that isn't tied to a specific course. The exam covers many different content areas and is quite rigorous. Similarly, most states require initial-certification teacher candidates to take a content-knowledge exam such as PRAXIS™ II or one developed by the state.

Portfolios — collections of artifacts that candidates select to document competencies and learning or work samples — also can cut across semesters and courses. Portfolios are designed to show growth over time and provide an excellent snapshot of what program graduates can do. To alleviate data-storage problems, some programs now use electronic portfolios to gather and store artifacts. Regardless of format, portfolios can be excellent sources of data for program evaluation.

Many programs in the health sciences or teacher education areas also require candidates to serve an internship or complete student teaching experience. Results from a practicum experience, in which a supervisor uses program criteria to evaluate the intern or candidate are useful for documenting program effectiveness. Demonstrating excellence on content knowledge assessments is only part of the story; candidates also must be able to apply that knowledge in a workplace setting. Assessments designed to measure such competency are important for professional evaluation. In the case of graduate programs, comprehensive exams and theses can be excellent ways to document student knowledge and competencies.

Assessments Related to a Specific Course

Coursework provides another source of data for program evaluation. Projects that require several weeks of work and represent the culmination of learning for a semester can be excellent choices as program-evaluation assessments. Sport law professors often conclude their courses with a mock trial, for example, and a facilities management course might require an in-depth analysis of an existing facility or ask candidates to design a new structure.

The problem with using course assessments is that faculty members must choose carefully which assessments to track or they will have more data than they can evaluate. One way to discriminate and select the best course assessments is to go back to the matrix developed in Step 3. If a course is listed as contributing significantly to candidate knowledge for a content area, it probably is a good source of program evaluation data. Faculty members should go back to the objectives and determine which assessments were used to document that the candidate met the objective and then put those assessments on the matrix to determine the standards or content areas for which each assessment provides documentation and/or data.

Figure 2.2. Sample Assessment Matrix

Course

Objective/Goals/ Outcomes	Assessment	Standard(s) or Element(s) Addressed
Candidates will demonstrate the ability to write a complete objective containing all three components of a lesson plan.	Written lesson plan.	NASPE Initial PETE National Standard 3, Element 3.2: Develop and implement appropriate goals and objectives that align with local, state and/or national standards.
Candidates will make adaptations to their lesson-plan content development for teaching diverse students.	Written lesson plan.	NASPE Initial PETE National Standard 3, Element 3.5: Plan and adapt instruction for diverse student needs, adding specific accommodations and/or modifications for student exceptionalities.

NASPE's Initial PETE National Standards lend themselves to tracking teacher candidate performance on each standard and element, because candidates need to meet only 28 elements under six standards. Exercise science and athletic training standards, on the other hand, don't lend themselves to the same level of tracking.

ACSM's General Population/Core: Exercise Prescription and Programming guidelines identify 45 different knowledge, skills and abilities on which to assess candidates. That's just one of many sections on which exercise science majors are expected to demonstrate satisfactory performance. For that reason, program faculty members likely will hold students accountable for meeting those standards within courses but won't track the number of students who meet each standard. The objectives listed in course syllabi are specific, and they each state a criterion for performance. For the purpose of program evaluation, exercise science or athletic training programs that use ACSM guidelines could track candidate performance on:

- Some type of national exam (e.g., ACSM certifying exam, National Strength and Conditioning exam), with the various sub-domain scores disaggregated.
- Candidate performance during an internship.
- Evaluation of candidates from employers who hire graduates, and candidate evaluation of the program.

These big-picture assessments probably will be most helpful for program evaluation.

When identifying assessments for evaluation, program faculty members should focus on big-picture concepts necessary for candidates graduating from a program and identify at least two ways to assess each, one of which could be the general-content exam. Having multiple assessments for each of the major concepts will allow for better documentation. A rule of thumb: Identify enough assessments to measure program success but not so many that the information is redundant. The fewer assessments that a program uses to track candidate learning, the easier it will be to compile and use the data. One way to have fewer assessments is to select big-picture assessments that address multiple standards or topics.

Teacher education programs may submit only eight assessments for NCATE SPA program reports. That doesn't mean that program faculty members may not use additional assessments to measure excellence for university or internal use; it just means that the extra assessments won't be included in the accreditation report.

Identifying assessments for program evaluation is an important part of the process. Without high-quality assessments, the program won't be able to gather data on candidate performance during the program. Chapter 4 explores the evaluation of the data gathered from these assessments as the final portion of program evaluation.

Selecting Assessments for a Program Report

Selecting good assessments is critical for a strong program report, regardless of whether or not the report will be submitted for an accreditation review. So, what does a good assessment look like? If an assessment addresses several competencies or standards, it should be considered as a potential program assessment. This section is designed to give some guidance for selecting good assessments and to identify common mistakes that program faculty members make when selecting assessments.

Using Sub-Scores From Content-Knowledge Tests to Document Standards

When giving the results of a content-knowledge test, it's important that program faculty members disaggregate the data to show how candidates as a group performed on the various topics or sub-areas. If the program reports the total score as a single entity, it won't be possible to determine candidate performance for the various sub-areas of content knowledge. By disaggregating the data, program faculty members can determine whether candidates have sufficient knowledge about motor patterns, biomechanical principles, physiology, etc.

Using GPA to Document Candidates' Content Knowledge

Program faculty members might use grade point average (GPA) in a course or set of courses that all candidates are required to take as an indicator of content knowledge. The problem with using GPA is that criteria used to assign grades tend to be relative, and different courses are graded with different levels of rigor. Variation also can occur among instructors teaching the same course. If a program uses GPA to document content knowledge, program faculty members must provide a brief description of the courses and a rationale for selecting that particular set of courses. They also must provide a rationale for how the courses align with specific SPA standards, as well as an analysis of grade data included in the submission.

If GPA is used as an indicator of content knowledge, every instructor teaching every course within the program should use the same scale when assigning grades. *Remember:* A program report is only as good as the data used to write it. If program faculty members are going to use GPA to indicate candidate learning, they must establish meaningful criteria for the grading scale.

The ultimate goal of a program review (beyond accreditation) is to improve the program's quality. It's difficult to glean much from a GPA; other sources of information about content knowledge usually are far more helpful. For those and other reasons, we strongly suggest that program faculty members use assessments other than GPA.

For those writing a NASPE SPA program report, we provide a comprehensive explanation of how to use GPAs as one of the assessments in Appendix A. Program faculty members should remember that they can use GPA for only one of the eight assessments in the NCATE program report. Other programs can use Appendix A as a model if they use GPA for program evaluation.

Align the Assessment With the Verb Used in the Standard or Goal

When program faculty members use national standards to develop a report, the verb used in the standard often is the key to matching an assessment with the standard or its element. If the standard simply requires a program to "document" content knowledge (e.g., knowing the systems of the body and what each one does), for example, then a written exam on the topic is sufficient. However, if the standard requires program candidates to "apply" the knowledge, then a written test is not the best way to assess application of knowledge and skills. Because it's very difficult, if not impossible, to write application questions on a written exam, it's much more appropriate to use hands-on/practical experience as a way for candidates to demonstrate the application of their knowledge. Course projects often require higher levels of thinking (e.g., synthesis, analysis, evaluation) and, thus, provide an excellent way to document candidates' higher levels of learning.

Program faculty members who develop their own standards should select a verb that represents the appropriate type of candidate learning. Words such as "understand" and "know" are impossible to measure and, therefore, should be avoided.

Use a Person of Authority to Document Candidate Performance

Several different types of assessment are useful in helping candidates become more competent professionals. Summative assessments given at the end of a course usually represent the candidate's final mastery of content. Not all types of assessment, though, should be used to document candidate performance for a program report. For example, peer assessments are excellent ways to increase learning in a class activity (e.g., as a formative assessment), but because they are completed by novice evaluators, they might lack reliability. Some peer evaluators might be reluctant to give low scores, which further decreases the value of the assessment.

Assessments should be meaningful and significant in high-stakes testing contexts (and program reports certainly are high-stakes). This means that a person of authority (e.g., course instructor, teaching assistant) should evaluate the candidates rather than a member of the class, and that the assessments should represent a comprehensive snapshot of candidate learning.

Ensure Reliability

To ensure that the data are reliable, program faculty members should have about 20 percent of the data checked by another person (inter-rater reliability) or by the same person (intra-rater reliability) at a later time. Although it's not necessary to cross-check data for a report not intended for accreditation, it's a good practice to follow. Cross-checking for reliability ensures that the data are accurate and provide information that's useful for making important program decisions.

Make Sure That You Have a Bona Fide Assessment

When looking at the assessments used for a course, it's important to remember that an assessment has two parts: the first is the task that is to be completed, and the second consists of the criteria used to evaluate the quality of the task (Morrow Jr., Jackson, Disch & Mood, 2010). Some people develop only a task and think that they've created an assessment. Without establishing a level of expectation for the level of quality that the candidate must demonstrate, the task is nothing more than an assignment or class requirement; it is not a tool for documenting candidate learning.

The criteria are very important, because they provide the performance expectations for the standards. Most standards written by accrediting agencies are "content standards" (broad, general statements of content) and don't specify the level of quality expected to satisfy the standard. Such a statement of quality is referred to as a "performance standard." Most accrediting agencies leave it up to individual programs to set the bar for candidate performance expectations. Typically, universities also allow programs to set their own criteria for candidates. It's very important for program faculty members to include the criteria so that candidates understand what is expected of them. At a minimum, they should define what is acceptable and unacceptable for candidate performance. Chapter 3 discusses the development of rubrics, which can be used for indicating levels of quality. Program faculty members need to remember that criteria show reviewers (either for program accreditation or for university requirements) the program's rigor.

Using Enough Assessments to Document Candidate Knowledge

When deciding how many assessments to include, the more documentation that program faculty members can provide, the more trustworthy the data will be. Using several assessments to evaluate the same element or standard is similar to the technique that a researcher would use when trying to triangulate data to arrive at a defensible decision about the data. For program evaluation, faculty members should consider triangulation of data when selecting assessments.

The data are important for documentation and to show trends, but — ultimately — the decisions made by the people interpreting the data are more important. And the first step in making good decisions is to make sure that the data on which those decisions are based are trustworthy (e.g., valid and reliable). The second step is to ensure that the person making the decision has enough information, from a variety of sources, to determine whether the candidate has, in fact, reached the criterion level needed to meet the standard. Only then can program faculty members have confidence in making a decision about a program's quality.

Because teacher education programs are limited to eight or fewer assessments for NCATE reports, program faculty members must be careful to select assessments that will provide optimal coverage of the standards and their elements. If an assessment provides substantial evidence, faculty members should, if possible, document candidate learning with two assessments. If the assessment provides only minor evidence, more documentation will be necessary.

One caveat: Some programs use assessments that are only remotely connected to the element being assessed. That practice can be counterproductive, because using several weak assessments can create unnecessary work for the faculty and staff members who compile the data. In the case of reports submitted for accreditation, this practice can cast doubt about program faculty members' level of knowledge about the standards and related elements. It might seem as though the program is tossing everything it can into the report rather than displaying a thorough understanding of what the standard means and providing appropriate evidence that addresses it. Best practice requires that program faculty members should list only those assessments that have the greatest relevance to the standard or element.

Conclusion

Selecting appropriate assessments to document candidate learning is an essential part of program evaluation. Strong assessments that are aligned with program outcomes are essential to improving program quality, because they provide meaningful data on which to make decisions. By following the steps and suggestions outlined in this chapter, program faculty members can select assessments that are meaningful and relevant to the program.

Chapter 3

Creating Rubrics for Professional Preparation Program Assessment

Many programs develop outstanding assessments for evaluating program quality but then fail to fully define the expectations for candidate performance. A good rubric is an essential part of an assessment because it defines the level of quality necessary to satisfy the intent of the assessment. This chapter focuses on writing analytic qualitative rubrics and provides examples of rubrics for various assessments. We note potential problems when developing rubrics and suggest ways to avoid them. The chapter concludes with some suggestions for developing high-quality rubrics for program evaluation.

Which Type of Rubric Should We Select?

Two common types of rubrics are used in education: (1) holistic rubrics, which evaluate the work as an entity; and (2) analytic rubrics, which are used to evaluate discrete parts of student work or performance. When a holistic rubric is used, a single score for the work is given, making it impossible for students to see which part of the work is done well and where improvements are needed. Holistic rubrics often are used for summative assessments for which only a final score is needed and students are not expected or given the opportunity to change it. If a work is given a low score because a part of it is substandard, the holistic rubric does not indicate where the weaknesses lie. When an analytic rubric is used, each of the parts is. When students look at the how the work was scored, they know where the strengths and weaknesses lie. Also, with an analytic rubric, some items can be weighted if they're more important to the overall assessment.

To illustrate the difference between the two types of rubrics: If you were judging a cake-baking contest, a holistic rubric would require you to give a single score to the cake, while an analytic rubric would require you to give separate scores for such aspects as taste, appearance, texture and moistness.

Analytic rubrics give program faculty members the capacity to disaggregate the data gleaned from an assessment, which is necessary for evaluating the subsections of each assessment. Thus, an analytic rubric provides the data that program faculty members need to evaluate the various characteristics or elements on an individual basis rather than collapsing all the parts into a single score, as is the case with holistic rubrics. We recommend using an analytic rubric for program reports because faculty members can use them to provide formative feedback to candidates who are completing the assessment and because of the program's need to disaggregate student data for reports.

There are two different types of analytic rubrics: (1) quantitative analytic rubrics, which use numbers and short phrases to distinguish among levels of performance; and (2) qualitative analytic rubrics, which use brief paragraphs to create verbal pictures of those differences. For the purpose of program reports, we prefer using qualitative analytic rubrics. This chapter, then, focuses on developing good qualitative analytic rubrics and provides several examples of them.

What Characterizes a Good Rubric?

A good rubric communicates expectations for learning and performance to program candidates, program faculty members and outside evaluators. Not all candidates have the same level of ability or put forth the same amount of effort, which means that the quality of their performances will vary. A good rubric helps faculty members recognize candidates who demonstrate outstanding skills and knowledge, distinguishing them from those who show less effort and/or ability. Also, a rubric helps program faculty members identify weaknesses in candidate performance, thus enabling program evaluators to identify possible gaps in the curriculum and areas that need more emphasis.

A good rubric consists of criteria that help faculty members judge the quality of a candidate's performance. Typically, a rubric's quality is determined by three characteristics:

1. Its ability to distinguish among levels of candidate performance.
2. Its clarity.
3. Its alignment with standards and/or program goals.

Ability to Distinguish Among Levels of Performance

For a rubric to be reliable, it's crucial that it establishes clear distinctions among the various levels of performance so that faculty members will apply it consistently. A poorly written rubric or one that lacks detail will cause issues with reliability because faculty members will have difficulty using it to distinguish among levels of candidate performance. Consider the differences between the rubrics found in Figures 3.1 and 3.2.

Figure 3.1. Rubric A for Behavior-Management Strategies

Category	Unacceptable	Acceptable	Target
Behavior-Management Strategies	Fails to identify behavior-management strategies.	Identifies some behavior-management strategies.	Identifies a sufficient number of behavior-management strategies so that students know the rules of the class.

Figure 3.2. Rubric B for Behavior-Management Strategies

Category	Unacceptable	Acceptable	Target
Behavior-Management Strategies	Has given little thought to planning the unit's organization.	Identifies several routines that will help organize students during the unit.	Describes a classroom-management plan to maximize on-task behavior.
	Rules and routines are general and are not related specifically to the unit's content or implementation.	States rules in a positive way, while noting appropriate consequences.	Encourages students to self-monitor behavior.
	Identifies a few behaviors that are appropriate and inappropriate. Management plan includes ineffective or inappropriate consequences.	Identifies several appropriate and inappropriate behaviors specific to the unit.	Identifies routines that will lead to a smoothly run unit of instruction. Designs rules in a way that encourages student self-management.
	Pays little attention to students' safety during the unit.	Specifies safety procedures that are aligned with school safety plans, while noting contingency plans.	Identifies appropriate and inappropriate behaviors and makes plans to instruct students on how those behaviors will be taught and encouraged.
	Uses several strategies that are weak and/or ineffective.		States safety procedures clearly, taking into account a variety of scenarios that may arise while implementing the unit.

The second example contains far richer descriptions about expectations for candidate performance when the candidate identifies behavior-management strategies for a unit plan assessment. The detail is helpful for candidates when completing the assignment; they can determine the program's expectations and what they must do to move their performance to a higher level. Also, the rubric in Figure 3.2 uses vocabulary from the program, which provides an indicator of quality that external reviewers use to determine program quality.

Some programs use quantity or frequency to distinguish among performance levels. For example, a program might indicate that an acceptable performance would require evidence of three management strategies, while a target level of performance would require evidence of four or more strategies. We urge caution here because, although the rubric's reliability will be high, its validity might be low. If the management strategies that the candidate lists are weak, a greater number of them won't improve the quality of the candidate's work.

In some instances, a number on a rubric is used to indicate consistency or accuracy. If, for example, a candidate shows the ability to take a blood pressure reading accurately (e.g., within a certain acceptable range of error) and consistently (e.g., three times in a row), that would be an acceptable use of numbers in a rubric to differentiate performance levels. Program faculty members must be sure that numbers are a valid way to distinguish levels of excellence before using them on a rubric.

Clarity

A good rubric should communicate expectations for performance in a clear and concise manner, and eliminate subjective judgment to the extent possible. Sometimes, rubrics contain vague terms such as "effort" or "sportsmanship" but fail to define what behaviors those terms are meant to represent.

The rubric in Figure 3.1 fails to identify the different performance levels, requiring those using it to apply subjective judgment. What is the candidate failing to identify? How many are "some"? The target level prescribes that a "sufficient number" be identified. Is the number the important element here, or is it that the strategies identified are effective? Generally, if several questions arise after reading the rubric, it lacks clarity.

In contrast, the rubric in Figure 3.2 contains more descriptors, but that's not the most important difference; it's that the descriptions and examples of what candidate performance on the assessment should look like at each level help clarify program expectations.

Another common error found on rubrics occurs when a rubric restates a description at each level but uses different words to indicate the level of rigor (e.g., "Identifies *some* behavior-management strategies" versus "Identifies a *sufficient number* of behavior-management strategies" versus "Identifies *several* behavior-management strategies"). Rubrics that restate the descriptor lack clarity and often require scorers to interpret a level of quality instead of spelling out that level themselves.

Alignment With Standards and/or Program Goals

Rubrics for program assessments should contain a direct link to, or be aligned with, either a standard or a program goal. The rationale for that is twofold: first, to ensure that all necessary elements or goals are addressed; and second, to keep the report as concise and succinct as possible by not including extraneous elements that lack relevance for program quality. Typically, this link is found in the rubric's descriptor. It's not necessary to use the element's exact wording to show alignment with it but anyone reading the rubric shouldn't need to guess what element or program goal the rubric is being used to assess.

Two examples follow: one for those writing NASPE SPA reports and a second for those writing other types of program-evaluation reports.

NASPE Program Report Example

Element 3.2 reads:

> Develop and implement appropriate (e.g., measurable, developmentally appropriate, performance-based) goals and objectives aligned with local, state and/or national standards. (NASPE, 2009)

To satisfy the intent of the element fully, an assessment would require teacher candidates to both develop the written objective in some type of planning document and then use the objective in some type of practicum experience. The rubric should require candidates to write the objective for a plan and then use the objective when teaching.

Exercise Science Example

Ability 1.7.34 from ACSM's Guidelines for Exercise Testing and Prescription prescribes that candidates should have the ability to:

Evaluate, prescribe and demonstrate flexibility exercises for all muscle groups.

That ability statement is quite complex and requires candidates to know the muscle groups associated with various joints of the body. Knowing the joints of the body is a prerequisite for completing Ability 1.7.34 and will be assessed indirectly during the assessment. Because this standard addresses an ability, a performance-based assessment (i.e., one that involves a candidate actually performing the evaluation, prescription and demonstration of flexibility exercises) is an excellent way to assess it. The rubric for the assessment task would focus on three areas: the candidate's ability to (1) evaluate the client's flexibility status, (2) prescribe flexibility exercises based on the client's needs and (3) demonstrate those exercises while teaching the client how to perform them.

The rubric should explore the accuracy of candidates' decisions in determining the client's status of flexibility and selecting exercises for the client. When demonstrating the exercises, candidates might be required not only to point out how to perform the exercises, but also to provide tips (e.g., "You should feel it work this muscle," or "You should feel the stretch here") for ensuring that the client performs them correctly when working without supervision.

Deciding Between Generalized Rubrics and Task-Specific Rubrics

After program faculty members have developed or identified the assessment, they must develop the criteria with which to evaluate the candidate's quality of work. They can take either of two approaches in writing the rubric. One approach is to write a generalized rubric that can be used for multiple assessments. The second approach is to write a task-specific rubric for each assessment. Each of those approaches comes with advantages and disadvantages. The next section provides more information about each approach.

Generalized Rubrics

Well-written generalized rubrics address the concepts that are important to the program (e.g., content standards and/or elements, program goals) and are appropriate for evaluating multiple assessments. One can think of a generalized rubric as a universal rubric, with descriptors that specify appropriate levels of performance regardless of the assessment with which the rubric is used. For example, if sport management program faculty members want to develop rubrics for the program goals or outcomes, they would begin by identifying what those outcomes are and then develop a rubric that describes the behaviors and competences that candidates should demonstrate when they meet program expectations. For example, budget-planning knowledge is used with many assessments or assignments; the generalized rubric is written to the universal concepts and competencies that program graduates should demonstrate. Similarly, exercise science or athletic training faculty members might write a generalized rubric that addresses protocols for demonstrating exercises for fitness improvement or rehabilitation.

In teacher education, the goals for a program are articulated in the PETE standards. When preparing an NCATE accreditation report, program faculty members might write a generalized rubric for each initial PETE standard or element. When developing a rubric for a specific assessment from the comprehensive generalized rubric, faculty members select the applicable standards and elements from the generalized rubric that apply to the assessment and then use those criteria or levels of performance to create the rubric; those not relevant are omitted. For example, the assessment might not address candidate fitness levels so that descriptors from NASPE's Initial PETE Standard 2's Element 2.2 — Achieve and maintain a health-enhancing level of fitness throughout the program — would not be included. This approach will work for teacher education and sport management programs. Exercise science faculty members would face a daunting task if they tried to write a generalized rubric for all of the required abilities, skill and knowledge statements.

Generalized rubrics are more difficult to develop; visualizing a desired performance or behavior outside the context of an assessment is more difficult than visualizing performance on a specific assessment. The advantage of using a generalized rubric is that, once it's written, faculty members won't need to develop additional rubrics for those descriptors or elements when they appear in other assessments. Figures 3.3 and 3.4 provide examples of generalized rubrics that could be used for multiple assessments.

Figure 3.3. Sample Generalized Rubric for NASPE Initial PETE Standard 4, Element 4.1

Descriptor	Unsatisfactory	Acceptable	Target
4.1: Demonstrates effective verbal and non-verbal communication skills across a variety of instruction formats.	Provides lengthy, unclear instructions. Uses primarily verbal explanations of the task. Describes the task in terms not easy to understand. Does not tell students the intent and/or purpose of the lesson. Offers mostly general feedback or feedback that is not related to the task being performed. Sometimes uses statements that indicate bias or lack of sensitivity to student differences.	Provides instructions that are easy to understand but takes a long time to deliver them. Describes tasks in a way that helps students understand what to do. States lesson objectives. Offers mostly specific feedback, but targets fewer than half of the students in the class. Communicates in ways that are free from bias. Shows sensitivity to individual differences.	Provides clear, concise instructions. Provides an understandable description of the task. Uses kinesthetic and visual cues along with verbal descriptions. States lesson objectives clearly for all three domains. Offers feedback that is specific and congruent. Encourages all students to do their best; has high performance expectations for all students.

Figure 3.4. Sample Generalized Rubric for Exercise Science or Athletic Training for Demonstrating and Teaching Exercises to Clients

Descriptor	Unsatisfactory	Acceptable	Target
Accurate demonstration of the skills.	Performs/ demonstrates the exercise incorrectly. Moves through the demonstration quickly, making it difficult for the client to learn the exercise.	Demonstrates the exercise correctly. Performs the exercise slowly for learning purposes and then at a regular pace so that the client has a clear idea of what the exercise looks like.	Meets the criteria in the "Acceptable" category, and also allows the client to perform the exercise along with the demonstration. Stops at key places during the demonstration to emphasize important parts of the exercise.
Provides correct information.	Uses incorrect terminology during the demonstration; gives erroneous or misleading information. Uses jargon rather than putting terms in layperson's language.	Provides accurate information about the exercise and uses correct terminology. Uses language that the client can understand.	Meets the criteria in the "Acceptable" category, and also explains the benefits of performing the exercise. Points out common errors and explains what to avoid.
Interaction with client.	Fails to give the client full attention (e.g., looks elsewhere, talks on cell phone, listens to iPod, talks with others). Sometimes leaves the client during the session. Does not supervise while the client performs the exercise.	Makes the client feel that his/her interests are the main focus of the session. Stays with the client to supervise the session.	Meets the criteria in the "Acceptable" category, and also starts the session promptly. Maintains eye contact with the client. Supervises the client closely to ensure that exercises are done correctly; requires sufficient repetitions to ensure the exercise's effectiveness.
Presentation skills.	Uses poor grammar; talks so that he/she is difficult to understand (e.g., mumbles, uses slang, words are hard to hear or understand). Gives too much information, slowing the pace of the session.	Speaks clearly, using proper grammar most of the time. Is easy to understand and uses age-appropriate language.	Meets the criteria in the "Acceptable" category, and also uses voice inflection to encourage the client. Adds variety to the session to make the time enjoyable and/or pleasant.

Task-Specific Rubrics

Task-specific rubrics are written for specific assessments. The person developing the rubric identifies those characteristics that a candidate completing the assessment should demonstrate and then writes descriptions of the performance levels to evaluate the quality of the work. Task-specific rubrics are easier to write, because the developer has an actual assessment in mind and then describes the levels of performance associated specifically with the assessment; there is no need to write the rubric at a universal level for multiple assessments. For example, a task-specific rubric would evaluate game play in badminton instead of game play for sport in general, or would evaluate a presentation during a mock trial instead of presentations in general. Figure 3.5 is part of a task specific rubric written for use with a mock trial.

One advantage of using task-specific rubrics is that they typically require less training than generalized rubrics to ensure reliable scoring because they tend to contain more detail specific to the assessments. Also, task-specific rubrics are easier for teacher candidates to use in self-assessing their work.

Figure 3.5. Sample of a Partial Task-Specific Rubric for a Mock Trial

Descriptor	Unsatisfactory	Acceptable	Target
Presentation of evidence	Presents evidence in a haphazard manner, making it difficult for others to follow. Uses filler words, making it hard to follow the intent of the evidence. Leaves it to the audience to determine links between the information presented and the relevance to the purpose of presenting the evidence.	Presents evidence systematically, using a logical order. Uses vocabulary that is at an appropriate level of difficulty and is easy to understand. Is purposeful in the presentation, without using filler words. Makes occasional links between the information/evidence presented and its relevance to the case.	Presents evidence systematically, using a logical order. Uses diagrams to help others gain meaning from the evidence. Presentation flows and is free from grammar errors and filler words. Uses voice inflection and pauses deliberately to emphasize key points. Establishes a clear link between the evidence and its relevance to the case. Emphasizes key points in a summary at the end of the presentation.

Using task-specific rubrics has its disadvantages, as well. It can take a lot of time to develop a rubric for the quality necessary for use in a high-stakes evaluation. Also, if the task-specific rubric is used by multiple people, training is required before use, to ensure consistent application of the criteria. In contrast, with a generalized rubric, faculty members are trained to use one rubric.

Developing a Task-Specific Rubric

Although the process of developing a task-specific rubric is similar to developing a generalized rubric, a task-specific rubric usually is easier to develop because it's linked to a single assessment. For that reason, we begin by explaining how to develop a task-specific rubric.

Step 1. Brainstorm a list. Before starting to write a rubric, program faculty members should consider what the assessment is meant to evaluate. For example, if the rubric is not aligned to the assessment's purpose, the assessment's validity will be compromised severely or even negated. If the rubric is designed to assess presentations during a mock trial (Figure 3.5), then program faculty members should brainstorm ideas about what makes a presentation good and what a bad presentation looks like. While brainstorming, the rubric developers should try to envision what the performance or product should look like and identify those characteristics, as well as defining potential errors or misunderstandings that detract from the quality of candidate performance.

Step 2. Combine similar ideas. After brainstorming the initial list of desirable qualities for the targeted performance or product, rubric developers must determine whether some of the ideas listed represent the same construct or concept. In some instances, words from the brainstorm list might represent different levels of the same idea. In Step 2, rubric writers group the words developed in Step 1 so that topics or concepts for the assessment are developed. They then — in Step 3 — will use those groupings to develop descriptors. It's important to remember that too many items to evaluate can make the rubric difficult to use. An ideal number is five to eight groups of words. If a rubric seems to have more than that, rubric developers should take another look at the grouping and see whether other combinations are possible. A rubric should have enough descriptors to make it thorough but not so many as to make it cumbersome to use.

Step 3. Identify descriptors for the rubric. A descriptor is the name given to the key points or categories that the assessment will evaluate. In Step 3, the writers identify a word or group of words that represents a concept that the cluster of words from Step 2 represents. For the rubric on demonstrations *(see Figure 3.4),* the descriptors include demonstrating the skills accurately, providing the correct information, interacting with the client and exhibiting effective presentation skills.

Step 4. Determine the number of performance levels that the program will use to evaluate candidates' performance on the assessment. Each rubric should contain at least two candidate performance levels: acceptable and unacceptable. The "acceptable" level should reflect the minimum level of performance that a candidate can demonstrate and still pass the assessment. Most programs add a third level to the rubric to describe a "target" behavior, or a level of performance that faculty members want all candidates to achieve. A target level tells candidates where the program would prefer their level of performance to be. It also encourages candidates to strive to surpass the minimum performance required to pass the assessment.

If rubric developers add a "target" performance level to the rubric, does that create enough levels? Wiggins (1998) recommends also adding a level to describe performance *above* the target level. Candidates rarely achieve this level, but it does provide a way of recognizing candidates who exceed expectations and demonstrate truly exemplary skills or abilities. If desired, faculty members can add more levels, depending on the program's philosophy and the desire to further delineate levels of performance. Some programs, for example, might write a rubric with five performance levels, to describe candidate performance at each of the grading levels (A, B, C, D and F). Rubric developers should keep in mind that the rubric's reliability decreases with the addition of each performance level because the difference between levels becomes less distinct. Determining the number of levels to use in the rubric is left to the discretion of program faculty members.

Step 5. Develop the rubric. In this step, rubric developers actually create the rubric by writing descriptions of the various levels of performance for each of the descriptors. The list of words generated in Step 1 is a valuable resource when beginning to write the rubric. Developers should also pay close attention as to whether the descriptors accurately reflect the desired levels of candidate performance for each of the descriptors. This step is more difficult to complete by oneself; working in teams of at least two people can help in developing the wording that best describes the desired level of performance.

Step 6. Pilot the rubric. The next step is to pilot the rubric on a low-stakes assessment (i.e., one that doesn't have a large impact on a candidate's grade or future standing in the program). A pilot administration of the assessment and rubric will reveal problems that developers could not have anticipated when developing the rubric. As a test of validity, the best students should receive the highest scores. If that's not the case, developers should revise the rubric.

Step 7. Revise the rubric. Faculty members with experience in writing rubrics expect to revise them after an initial use. Pilot-testing the rubric will reveal problems with it, and the subsequent revision will help ensure that, going forward, the rubric will be of higher quality. When revising the rubric after the pilot administration, it's important that developers look at the descriptors to ensure that all of the desired characteristics and knowledge are addressed. Developers might find that combining some descriptors streamlines and, thus, improves the rubric's quality, or that more descriptors are needed. During the revision, it's important to look at the levels of performance on the rubric and ask these questions: "Are the levels so demanding that even the best candidates failed to reach the target level?" "Are the levels of performance expectations so low that all students reached the target level of performance with minimal effort?" "Are some descriptions of the levels unclear?" The responses to those questions will provide further ideas for improving the rubric's quality.

Developing a Generalized Rubric

The process for developing a generalized rubric is very similar to that for a task-specific rubric; the main differences are in the first 4 steps. The following explains how to develop a generalized rubric.

Step 1: Identify the concepts or descriptors. A generalized rubric is written to evaluate concepts rather than a specific assessment; therefore, when developing a generalized rubric, program faculty members must begin by identifying those concepts. Faculty members can use generalized rubric to evaluate many assessments. If a field or discipline has specific elements like those found in PETE or health, a good strategy would be to start with the standards and elements. In the case of sport management, when the program is expected to generate the concepts important for the program, those concepts must be identified. Both exercise science and sports medicine have very specific and comprehensive program requirements for candidate abilities and skills. In writing a generalized rubric for either of those two content areas, writers would develop a list of concepts that capture the essence of the details that a program aspires to achieve with its candidates, rather than developing levels of performance for each of the abilities, skills and knowledge. Figure 3.4 provides an example of a generalized rubric that program faculty members could use for multiple assessments.

Step 2. Brainstorm a list of behaviors. In this step, rubric developers look at the concepts and write descriptions of the desired behaviors, as well as potential errors or misunderstandings if the concept is not met. While brainstorming, developers should try to envision what the performance or product should look like for a variety of assessments.

Step 3. Determine the number of performance levels that the program will use to evaluate candidates' performance on the assessment. The work for this level is described under Step 4 for developing a task-specific rubric. Please refer to that section next.

Step 4. Write the rubric. Using the list of behaviors identified in Step 2, rubric developers now must decide what level of performance those behaviors represent on the rubric. When completing this step, developers should ensure that the descriptions for the various levels represent clear differences in performance so that those using the rubric will be able to use it reliably. In this step, the rubric is written.

The process used to develop Step 5 (pilot) and Step 6 (revision) is the same one used in Steps 6 and 7 for task-specific rubrics.

Other Factors to Consider When Writing Rubrics

This section provides a brief overview of some other factors to consider when developing rubrics.

How High Should Programs Set the Bar?

A good rubric helps faculty members communicate clearly where the bar for candidate performance is set when writing either external or internal reports. For performance-based assessments, the rubric is the vehicle for communicating with others about the level of rigor that the program requires of its candidates. Typically, external reviewers will question assessments that require little effort or that set the performance bar for "acceptable" at a low level. The ultimate goal for any program is to produce highly skilled and knowledgeable graduates; the goal of the review should be to improve program quality. Setting the bar at an appropriate level of difficulty is critical to ensuring a high-quality program.

Ensuring Reliability

Because many people will be using a program's rubric, training is absolutely necessary to make sure that everyone who uses it interprets the criteria in the same manner. Some faculty members give greater importance to some descriptors than other descriptors, thereby weighting them. If descriptors are weighted, all faculty members must apply the weighting system in the same way.

A common error occurs when faculty members score candidate work based on their perceptions of candidate performance rather than following the descriptions of performance found on the rubric. In other words, they expect a level of performance from a candidate because they know the candidate from other venues and then award that level without actually applying the rubric's descriptions of quality. When possible, the person who scores the performance or product should be neutral, harboring no preconceptions or expectations.

Assuming that the course instructor is the person who will score the assessment, another faculty member should review some — 10 percent to 20 percent — of the assessments to ensure that the data are reliable. Faculty members must set the desired agreement percentage before conducting the reliability check. (Agreement on 80 percent of the materials evaluated often is used to represent an acceptable standard for reliability). It's best if the reviewer conducting the reliability check has little, if any, prior knowledge of the candidates; that's when judgment about a performance is most likely to be accurate.

Considering Validity

With projects and other types of performance-based rubrics, the assessment often requires candidates to demonstrate the exact behaviors required for meeting program goals or standards. Good validity means that the assessment has great potential to yield high-quality data about candidate performance. Program faculty members can establish validity by having several neutral faculty members (those external to the program either from elsewhere in the university or from other universities) check the alignment between the assessment and rubric. There are other ways to statistically establish validity, but they are beyond the scope of this publication. Program faculty members should keep in mind that, if an assessment is valid, the candidates who perform the best on the assessment should perform well consistently on other assessments designed to measure the same construct.

Another point to remember is that the rubric must target the right items or the assessment won't provide a valid measure of what it's intended to measure. Here's an example to illustrate the point: A professor designed an assessment that required candidates to use content knowledge to develop and deliver a presentation. Although the assessment had great potential to evaluate candidate content knowledge on the topic, the rubric was focused on candidates' presentation skills: quality of PowerPoint slides, clarity of speaking, grammar, professional dress, etc. If the assessment had been designed to assess candidates' presentation abilities, the rubric would have been valid, but it didn't allow the evaluator to make valid decisions regarding candidate ability and knowledge of content, thus rendering the assessment an inappropriate measure of content knowledge.

Eliminating Bias

Program faculty members should eliminate any bias (e.g., racial, ethnic, gender, body-type, disability-based, cultural) when writing rubrics to assess candidate performance. In some instances, the use of pejorative language to describe potential performance interjects bias. For example, a rubric might make a statement that assumes that the candidate maintains a healthy weight. Some assessments might contain bias if they give privilege to or require one gender to do something that the other gender isn't required to do. In a mock trial, for example, the role of judge should not automatically be assigned to a male.

Bias also can occur when an assignment requires candidates to use resources to which some of them don't have access. Another example: Many campuses have computer labs where candidates can print assignments, but candidates using the labs might not have access to color printers to embellish graphs and tables, thus giving those candidates with their own color printers an advantage. Program faculty members should review assessments and rubrics to ensure that they are free of bias.

Using Exemplars

Exemplars — examples of previously scored candidate work — are used to help ensure consistent scoring. By viewing exemplars, a scorer can see examples of different levels of performance for candidate work and note how they were scored. In a sense, the exemplar calibrates the rubric (e.g., this paper represents a 3, this represents a 2). When using candidate work as an exemplar, program faculty members must remove the candidate's name and any other identifying characteristics and secure the candidate's permission before using it.

Suggestions for Writing Quality Rubrics

Writing rubrics is not a simple endeavor. This section offers suggestions intended to make the writing process a little easier.

Avoid Hyper-General Rubrics

A hyper-general rubric contains minimal information and leaves much of the judgment to the scorer instead of providing sufficient guidance and direction *(see Figure 3.6)*. Often, rubric writers use a single word to differentiate between performance levels and then neglect to define that word.

Figure 3.6. Example of a Hyper-General Rubric

	Unsatisfactory	**Acceptable**	**Target**
Demonstration of an exercise for a client results in the client's being able to perform the exercise correctly.	Following the demonstration, the client is <u>unable</u> to perform the exercise.	Following the demonstration, the client is <u>able</u> to perform the exercise.	Following the demonstration, the client is <u>able</u> to perform the exercise <u>well</u>.

The person using this rubric has little information for judging the quality of the candidate's work. Changing an adjective or a few words from one performance level to another isn't enough to fully describe the difference between the levels. The description of quality in a rubric should provide the person using it with guidance and clear criteria to ensure reliable scoring.

Rubrics Should Describe a Behavior, Not the Absence of One

Some rubric writers have difficulty describing an undesirable or unacceptable behavior in a rubric. In many cases, the rubric states simply that the candidate didn't demonstrate the behavior but then fails to describe what the student or client *did* demonstrate. Consider the difference between the following two descriptions of "unacceptable" in Figure 3.7, below.

Figure 3.7. Descriptions of Unacceptable Performance for NASPE Initial PETE Standard 3, Element 3.7

NASPE Element	Example A	Example B
3.7. Demonstrate knowledge of current technology by planning and implementing learning experiences that require students to use technology appropriately to meet lesson objectives.	Candidate fails to demonstrate the use of technology while planning and implementing learning experiences that require students to use technology appropriately to meet lesson objectives.	Technology selected for the lesson is inappropriate for the age of the student or fails to align with the lesson's goals. Technology is used in a superficial manner, unrelated to instruction or in a way that actually might impede student learning. The use of technology might have been planned, but the candidate failed to fully implement the plan because of managerial issues or insufficient resources.

When describing the "unsatisfactory" level, faculty members must remember that some type of behavior will occur; the goal is to describe what unsatisfactory behavior looks like. Common errors or misunderstandings usually provide good sources of descriptive terms for the "unsatisfactory" level. Complete descriptions also help candidates when they self-assess, by identifying the behaviors to avoid.

Match the Verb to Determine What's Expected of the Candidate

If a standard requires candidates to do more than one thing, it typically is aimed at moving instruction from one knowledge level to a higher level of learning, such as requiring candidates to apply the knowledge. In the previous exercise science/athletic training example *(see Figure 3.4)*, the candidate was expected to evaluate, prescribe and demonstrate to satisfy the assessment. A basic knowledge set is inherent in the standard, but Ability 17.34 requires candidates to evaluate a client's needs, which represents a higher-level thinking skill, more than mere basic knowledge of exercises. Candidates also must prescribe the flexibility exercises, thus requiring them to make decisions when selecting an exercise that is appropriate to the client's needs. If the rubric in this example describes only the behaviors for evaluating the client's needs, then it hasn't met the intent of the requirement.

Similarly, looking at Figure 3.7, Standard 3 relates to planning and implementing instruction. The rubric must examine candidates' ability to both plan and implement; either item alone will not satisfy the intent of the standard. By looking at the verbs in the standards and elements, program faculty members can determine what they expect teacher candidates to do. Stated simply, the rubric must align with the intent of the standard before it can document that the standard or element was met.

Use the Same Rubrics for Multiple Purposes

Rubrics are not easy to write and can be time-consuming to use for scoring candidate work. Whenever possible, program faculty members should develop rubrics and then use them for teaching, program evaluation and/or report preparation. That way, faculty members would need to write only one rubric, and candidate performance would be assessed only once (with the exception of re-scoring by another reviewer for reliability-check purposes).

Work With an Assessment Team to Develop Rubrics

It's difficult for one person to write a comprehensive, perfect rubric. It's very helpful to review rubrics as a group before using them, to clarify wording and to ensure that clear differences separate the levels. One strategy for doing that is to have assessment team members review the rubric and state expectations either in writing or orally, using their own words. These interpretations are then compared to the writer's original intent for the rubric and appropriate changes are made.

Requiring people to interpret the rubric can reveal inappropriate or confusing words. Program faculty members might use terminology differently. Multiple people should review rubrics for clarity and possible omissions (e.g., items missed when the rubric was written) before using them with candidate work.

Expect to Revise Your Rubrics

Good rubrics will evolve over time. Even program faculty members with a lot of experience writing rubrics go back and revise them. Use the rubric the first time with candidates in a course to see how well they perform. After using a rubric for course assignments, the instructor should make revisions immediately, while the necessary changes are fresh in his or her mind. Using a rubric for a course assignment actually serves as a pilot administration of the assessment (so long as the assignment does not comprise a major part of the course grade).

A rubric is ready for use in a high-stakes assessment if it required only limited revisions during the pilot. If a significant number of revisions were needed, we suggest that program faculty members use the assessment and rubric again in a low-stakes situation to determine whether the changes made improved the ability to evaluate candidate performance. Note that data collection for a report should not begin until the rubric is ready for use.

Use Previous Candidate Work to Write the Rubric

If the instructor has implemented the assessment previously, he or she can use examples of candidate work to establish the difference between levels. Sorting candidate work into levels of quality (e.g., acceptable, unacceptable and target) and then determining the differences in candidate performance between the piles (i.e., why a paper was placed in one pile instead of another) is a good way to develop a qualitative rubric.

One way to accumulate candidate work to use in developing an analytic rubric is to use the assessment in a pilot or low-stakes situation and then evaluate it with a checklist or quantitative analytic rubric. The instructor can require candidates to complete all parts of the assessment, with completion being the primary goal. The next time the instructor uses the assessment, he or she will develop a qualitative analytic rubric based on students' previous performance on the pilot.

Developing a Bridge Rubric

Some teacher education programs must use a unit rubric (e.g., one developed for an entire college or teacher education department) for certain assessments. The most common example of that is the rubric used to evaluate student teaching. If a program must use a unit-level rubric, faculty members can write a bridge rubric (i.e., one that bridges between the unit-level rubric and one more appropriate for the program) that shows the relationship between the PETE standards and the requirements of the unit-level rubric.

Usually, unit-level rubrics are generic and, theoretically, can be used in any teacher education program. Typically, unit-level rubrics are more applicable to a classroom than a gymnasium. The bridge rubric can expand on behaviors that might not be necessary for classroom instruction but are important for teaching a gymnasium. If program faculty members are required to report student teaching data to the unit using the unit-level rubric or, in the case of a faculty member from another program supervising student teachers for a physical education program, a bridge rubric can provide the necessary interpretation so that reviewers can see the relationship between the two and ensure that the candidates are required to perform all the elements specified in the PETE standards.

Checklist for a Good Rubric

We offer the following list of questions to help program faculty members develop rubrics for program evaluation. The checklists are designed to provide guidelines for ensuring that all of the necessary components are addressed when developing a rubric.

Yes	No	
___	___	Does the rubric feature clear distinctions between the levels of performance?
___	___	Does it align with standards and elements for the program?
___	___	Is the rubric written clearly so that other members of the program can paraphrase expectations after reading them?
___	___	Is it free from bias (e.g., gender, culture, race, ethnicity)?
___	___	Does the rubric describe the behaviors or indicators of unacceptable performance?
___	___	Does it contain the correct descriptors for the assessment used so that the desired content or performance is addressed (e.g., is the rubric valid)?
___	___	Are the descriptions on the rubric rich enough to allow the scorer to develop a mental picture of the expected performance or behavior?

Conclusion

Writing rubrics for a program is not an easy task. However, if faculty members put in the time and effort required for developing high-quality rubrics, collecting and reporting data for a program will be less difficult. Good rubrics help faculty members identify areas of strength and areas that could be improved, paving the way for ensuring that the program grows and improves.

Chapter 4
Using Data for Program Improvement

Many programs develop good assessments and rubrics to measure candidate performance based on the standards, but some stumble when using data to track program success. It's not possible, nor is it necessary, to track all the data that a candidate generates while completing a program. It *is* important, however, to save the right data and to make those data readily available to program faculty members. This chapter provides some guidelines for developing a system for storing and retrieving the data that are critical to documenting candidate performance, and concludes with a section on how program faculty members can use data to evaluate the quality of a program.

Collecting, Organizing & Retrieving Program Data

When you stop to think about it, effective programs have a lot of information about their candidates. Candidates are required to complete tests, projects, portfolios and other documents that are used to ensure their competency in the courses required to complete the major. While taking advanced or higher-level courses, candidates develop specific skills for a practicum or field setting, including the ability to write lesson plans, fitness plans for clients or rehabilitation programs for patients. Many programs require practicum work (e.g., student teaching, internships, lab experience), which provides a wealth of information about candidates' ability to apply knowledge.

Gathering data is not the difficult part of candidate or program evaluation; rather, the difficulty arises in deciding which data are needed for program evaluation and review, creating a systematic way of storing all of that information and developing a system for retrieving those data efficiently. We offer the ideas that follow to help develop that plan.

Organize the System Around the Candidates

If the system is organized around the candidates, it will be much easier to access data for reports. Each candidate should have a profile in the system so that program-performance information can be entered systematically. Each candidate should have some type of identification number, such as the one most universities assign candidates. A data-storage program such as ACT!, Goldmine or Excel can provide the platform for building the database. If the software selected is compatible with both MS Word and Excel, it's fairly easy to add information to candidates' profiles.

Gather Demographic Information on Candidates

Demographic information about candidates is very useful when creating reports, particularly when the college or university asks for a report on program diversity, retention or other issues. A list of demographic items might include but not be limited to age, gender, GPA when admitted to the university, GPA when admitted to the program, SAT scores (or GRE if for a graduate program), ethnicity, whether the candidate lives at home or independently, number of hours worked while taking courses, etc. Some of the information is available from university sources, while other information must come from the candidate. If possible, candidates should enter the information electronically, putting it directly into the database. That process will help cut down on human data-entry error and will save time. If another person enters the information into the database, program faculty members must take measures to ensure its confidentiality and accuracy. **Remember:** *Collecting candidates' demographic information can be useful, but it must not invade candidates' privacy.*

Enter Information Regularly

A database that is kept current will make retrieving information for reports easy. After program faculty members decide what information to track, the program should commit to entering the data at the end of each semester. If the program uses the same rubric for grading in a course and for tracking program data, program faculty members will need to evaluate the assessment only once. If program faculty members use one rubric for grading an assignment/assessment for a course and a different rubric to score it for program data (e.g., a task-specific rubric written for the course and a generalized rubric written to the standards), they will need to score the assignment/assessment a second time.

Track More Assessments Than Needed

This suggestion will cause many people to groan. Keeping track of candidate information or program data for an external review can be laborious, and the thought of keeping track of more information than necessary can be almost painful. But the advantages of tracking more assessments than are needed for a report are worth the trouble. First, having more information will be helpful when making decisions about the program. For example, NCATE reports allow only eight assessments, which might not provide enough information to actually increase any program's quality and to track changes accurately. Faculty membership can change; with new faculty members come new ways of doing things. Additional assessments can help reveal more subtle changes in the program that might not be apparent from the assessments designated for an accreditation report.

The choice about which assessments to track for program evaluation should not be dictated by an accrediting agency, even though some agencies do require certain types of assessments. Rather, program faculty members must determine what assessments are needed to monitor program quality.

A second reason for tracking additional assessments is to provide for more effective reporting. Having additional assessments allows program faculty members the luxury of being able to select the most meaningful ones for documenting program and candidate quality. Additional assessments also build in flexibility; if program faculty members decide to change the assessments used for the report, one of the other assessments being entered into the database might provide a good substitute. If standards for certification or accreditation change, program faculty members will be ahead of the game if they have gathered information on areas not previously required for an accreditation report.

For evaluation purposes, program faculty members will want to look at data trends. It will be easier for them to identify trends if they have collected data for the same assessment over at least two semesters. Data collected over a longer term will reveal trends more accurately and, thus, will help program faculty members determine whether a data set reflects programmatic or curricular changes accurately, or is an anomaly.

If data are used from a course that has different majors enrolled (e.g., Introduction to the Allied Health Profession), department faculty members should consider developing a way to disaggregate the data by programs to provide the most useful information for the various programs. Also, they should not use data from elective courses for accreditation reports, because not every student is required to take the course.

Create a System for Tracking the Data

While programs should have a central location for storing data, not all faculty members need or even should have full access to or the ability to edit the information. Faculty members should be able to input information from their own courses, but they shouldn't have the ability to make changes to the master data input system. Making changes to the system should be the responsibility of a single person. Many of us have worked with a well-meaning faculty member who wanted to make something better, overestimated his/her technology skills, and messed up the system for everyone else. The information used to evaluate programs is too critical to risk having someone accidentally delete a file or inadvertently create inaccuracies.

The person who has ultimate control over the data must make sure that he or she is not the only person who knows how the system works, in case he or she leaves at some point. Other program faculty members also must know how to access the data.

We suggest that programs use data-storage software that's available commercially. Typically, information technology staff members have basic programming skills and can create simple databases. Such custom databases, though, can create problems. A large university, for example, encountered problems when a programmer who was in charge of data entry left for a position at another university. That person's successor lost much of the data because it couldn't be retrieved. The university could have avoided the problem by requiring the programmer to use a commercially available program or by having other personnel also trained on the system.

Also, program faculty members should ensure that all data are backed up on an external hard drive or system. If the computer on which data are stored falters or crashes, data might be lost. Backing up data at another location is just common sense.

Develop Logs to Track Changes in the Program

When changes occur in a program, candidate performance results can change, as well. The addition of new faculty members can result in certain program content being emphasized or de-emphasized. Course-scheduling differences (e.g., regular semester versus an intense, shortened summer term), and the use of electronic portfolios or online grading are just some examples of changes that can affect the quality of candidate work and assessment data.

Logs of program changes can be useful when looking at trends in assessment data. Without these logs, faculty members can forget the exact year or date that something occurred or when they implemented some new technique. Logging program changes alleviates the need to rely on the memories of busy faculty members.

Keep Copies of Candidates' Work

Although storage can be an issue, program faculty members should keep some hard copies of candidates' work at the various levels of performance (e.g., unacceptable, acceptable, target). Once names and other identifying marks are removed, these records can become candidate artifacts for exhibit rooms when external reviewers conduct site visits, or can become exemplars for scoring program assessments.

Program faculty members also can scan hard copies of candidates' work and store the documents electronically to avoid storage and space issues. It's important, however, to keep a log of the files so that they can be retrieved when needed. Marked-up hard copies can provide examples of feedback to students and also can help faculty members who are working on post-tenure reviews or promotion and/or tenure dossiers.

Document Affective Domain Learning

While meaningful for use in program change, data regarding candidates' dispositions (e.g., attitudes, perceptions, feelings) can be difficult to obtain. Some programs evaluate candidates' dispositions using a rubric at regular intervals across key courses. Candidates' perceptions also provide important information about the affective domain. Surveys can reveal candidates' attitudes and perceptions about topics that are important to the program (e.g., work habits, work ethics, attitudes toward change and receiving feedback from supervisors).

Candidates can complete surveys electronically, saving data-entry time and eliminating the danger of human transcription errors. Electronic surveys about perceptions (e.g., about working with students or clients with disabilities connected with a practicum or clinical experience) can be automated and sent when candidates complete certain courses. That eliminates another potential human error: forgetting to administer the survey when life becomes too hectic or when a course changes instructors. Assessing candidates' dispositions and perceptions about the program provides information important to making program changes.

Although it's difficult to develop ways to assess the affective domain, the data from these assessments add an important dimension to the program evaluation.

Use Full-Time Faculty to Teach Courses in Which Accreditation Data Are Gathered

Although it's not always possible, employing full-time faculty members for courses in which key program assessments are administered is a good idea. Here are three reasons why:

1. Programs need consistency in when key assessments are administered and reports are written. Consistency is much more likely with a permanent faculty member than with someone who is new to or possibly transient to the program. It's nearly impossible to ensure consistency when the course instructor changes every year or every semester.
2. A part-time or temporary instructor might not be aware of the need to administer an assessment or might assign it very late in the term, thus failing to give students adequate opportunity to complete it with a sufficient degree of quality.
3. A full-time faculty member will tend to have a greater commitment or buy-in to program improvement.

We recognize that part-time or adjunct faculty members can be excellent teachers. However, gathering data for key program assessments is far too important for state approval and/or accreditation purposes and shouldn't be left to a part-time employee.

Evaluating the Data

Once the data have been gathered, it's time to take the most exciting step: examining the data to evaluate program quality. Examining program data is similar to analyzing data from a research study. In a sense, program evaluation is a type of research … research that can lead to program improvement. We offer the following suggestions for evaluating the data generated from program assessments.

Plan to Examine the Data as a Faculty

After gathering all the information, it's a good idea for program faculty members to evaluate candidate work as a group. Faculty members should start by looking at each assessment and the results. It can be useful for course instructors to reflect on their courses and think about the ways that candidates approached the assessments.

Instructor reflections are not meant to offer excuses for candidate performance but, rather, should provide insight and ideas for ways to strengthen the course. In some courses, a change as simple as the order in which topics are addressed can affect overall candidate performance.

The quality of candidates can vary from year to year, with one group being very strong and the next group being of much lower ability. Large class size also can hinder candidates' opportunities to interact in class and affect the way time is allocated during practicum work.

Program faculty members should allocate enough time to evaluate the data — honestly and with an eye toward reversing undesirable trends — considering all factors that can affect learning. They should meet at least once a year to discuss what program improvements the data might indicate.

Put the Data in a Format That Shows Trends

Trends should start to emerge the second time an assessment is administered or used. Data should be arranged so that faculty members can evaluate performance in a logical sequence, perhaps chronological. It's very difficult to evaluate qualitative data, so it's wise to add a numeric value to data (e.g., score the data with a rubric) so that program faculty members can detect trends. It's easier to detect differences when data are measurable.

Program faculty members must separate or disaggregate the data to show trends. Looking at the sections of data will provide a better sense of where candidates are showing improvement or decline. Some assessments provide disaggregated data to the program. For example, the Praxis™ II or a content-knowledge exam often shows data by the various topics and categories assessed.

Often, it's useful to examine candidate work from a variety of perspectives to understand where weaknesses are occurring. For example, one program faculty member evaluated the use of assessments by teacher candidates during the student teaching experience. Although the lesson plan overview identified an assessment component within the lesson plan, further investigation revealed that candidates had not allocated enough time in the lesson to administer the assessments, nor did they provide an example of the assessment given to students. An analysis of the lesson objectives revealed that candidates were confused about lesson focus and, therefore, were not conducting the assessments because they didn't know what they were supposed to assess. Such unpeeling — much like one would do to an onion — sometimes is necessary to show where candidate learning is breaking down.

Some program faculty members try to perform a statistical analysis of the data to show differences. A statistical analysis would be counterproductive in programs with a small number of candidates, because major differences or changes would be necessary before they would become statistically significant. In those instances, graphing data or using charts to look at trends might be a better approach.

If an assessment is intended to document several standards or elements, it should be designed so that program faculty members can disaggregate data specific to a designated standard or element. If changes occurred in administering the assessments, program faculty members should look at program logs to determine whether those changes could account for any resulting differences or data trends.

Grouping data according to program phases (i.e., decision points) also provides a good way to review the information. One might group the phases as follows: Phase I, university core curriculum; Phase II, content knowledge; Phase III, applied content knowledge; Phase IV, student teaching, internship or field placement. By grouping the data according to phases of the program, faculty members can determine which program areas are strongest and where change might be warranted.

Make Changes Gradually

After reviewing the data, faculty members might have several ideas for improving the program's quality. We suggest implementing only a few changes at any one time to allow program faculty members to evaluate the impact before enacting more changes. Just as one shouldn't change too many variables during a research study, changing too many program or curriculum variables at once can interfere with faculty members' ability to determine what, if anything, is making a difference in the quality of candidate performance. If several changes are needed, we suggest that they be implemented in stages, so that program faculty members can determine the impact of each change.

When making staged changes to a program, program faculty members should identify those program/curriculum variables that they think would make the most significant difference and change those items first. Program faculty members can evaluate subsequent changes the following year and then implement the next series of changes.

If possible, program faculty members should consider making temporary changes until they can determine whether the changes affect candidates' learning. Sometimes, programs make dramatic curriculum changes only to find that the changes didn't address the problem or improve program quality. Instead of making curriculum changes, it might be wise to consider substituting a course without making a permanent change. After the course is offered, faculty members can determine the impact of the change. That "pilot" approach can ensure accurate catalog information while providing additional supporting evidence for future, more permanent curriculum changes.

Conclusion

Using data to drive decisions about program change is prudent and educationally sound. Educators can be guilty of jumping on bandwagons and implementing new ideas before undertaking any type of systematic evaluation of the change. In this chapter, we provided some strategies for developing a structure for comprehensive program evaluation and then storing data that have the potential to provide meaningful information for program improvement. The best approach for gathering program evaluation data is to save the most important data, provide an efficient way to enter the information into the database and include a retrieval system that allows program faculty members to examine the data in a meaningful way.

Chapter 5

'Unpacking' the National Standards for Initial PETE

This chapter targets "unpacking" standards specific to PETE programs. However, the strategies apply to all programs of study in which standards provide a framework for the curriculum, such as AAHE programs, teacher education programs and other academic programs for which standards are used. Faculty members in programs other than PETE programs might find it valuable to read through this chapter, even though the content knowledge required of degree candidates in those programs differs. Most teacher education programs have standards based on pedagogical content (e.g., planning, instruction, classroom management, assessment, reflection), so the example provided later in the chapter applies in that context. The section on how to "package" standards and elements when designing program assessments can benefit those in other kinds of programs, as well.

First, an explanation: "Unpacking the standards" means to clarify what the standards and associated elements mean, in addition to what skills, knowledge and dispositions (behaviors) candidates must be able to demonstrate to satisfy the standards. It also provides insight as to how to measure candidate success in meeting the standards and elements.

We begin with a brief overview of the 2008 National Standards for Initial PETE, and offer strategies to help program faculty members unpack those standards. Next, we outline the PETE standards and elements and provide a commentary that serves as an example of how the standards and elements might be unpacked. We conclude the chapter with a brief discussion of how to "package" the standards and elements when designing program assessments.

An Overview of the 2008 National Initial PETE Standards

NASPE's 2008 National Standards for Initial Physical Education Teacher Education consist of six standards and 28 associated elements (NASPE, 2009). PETE programs must meet all 28 elements to earn national recognition from the NASPE SPA. The performance-based standards and elements represent the knowledge, skills and dispositions needed to become an effective beginning physical education teacher.

The standards also reflect a longtime concern among PETE faculty: the notion of whether teacher candidates demonstrate a strong foundation in a variety of movement forms and physical activities. A second, somewhat related, issue refers to teacher candidates' levels of health-related fitness. Skillful movement and health-related fitness are now addressed in Initial PETE Standard 2: Skill-Based and Fitness-Based Competence. This substantive revision of the original, 2001 PETE standards was intended to bring about a more focused curricular effort targeting candidate skill and fitness-based competencies.

NASPE's PETE standards can serve many purposes, and they are the criteria by which PETE programs are evaluated for national accreditation. The standards also can provide a framework for driving the curriculum. Most important, the standards and elements set the bar for determining PETE program quality and the competency of its teacher candidates.

Strategies for Unpacking the Standards

Lund and Tannehill (2010) offer two key questions that program faculty members should ask when trying to unpack standards and associated elements:

1. What is the intent behind the standard?
2. How might one interpret the standard and its related elements?

Those two questions should be revisited often throughout the process of unpacking the standards. Program faculty members will find the following generic unpacking strategies useful in their interpretation of the standards. The strategies apply to any set of standards; they provide a guide to help faculty members interpret the intent behind the standards and/or elements accurately.

Strategy 1: Consider the verbs used within standards/elements. Dissect each standard and its elements. To do that, look first at the verbs used within the standard and/or elements. They indicate what the teacher candidate must be able to do; what behaviors must be evident. If, for example, an element states that candidates must "describe" and "apply" something, it means that candidates will have to *show* content knowledge and *apply* that knowledge in a manner that indicates they have met the standard. Addressing one or the other (knowledge or application) is not sufficient.

The verbs used within the standard and/or element also denote the level of learning as found in Bloom's Taxonomy of Learning Domains (e.g., knowledge versus application of content).

Strategy 2: Determine contexts/conditions. It's also necessary to determine the contexts or conditions in which the behavior is to occur. Consider Initial PETE Standard 2's Element 2.1 as an example:

> *Demonstrate personal competence in motor skill performance for a variety of physical activities and movement patterns.*

The context within which candidates are to demonstrate personal competence in motor skill performance is within "a variety of activities and movement patterns." "Variety," in this case, means several different types of physical activities, and "movement patterns" means performance related to fundamental movement/motor patterns (locomotor, non-locomotor and manipulative). Therefore, candidates must demonstrate personal competence in motor skill performance under both contexts. Again, demonstrating one or the other would not be enough to meet the intent behind the element.

Strategy 3: Search for terms such as 'and,' 'or,' 'and/or' and 'throughout.' Each term differs in meaning, based on how it's used within the standard or element. Consider these three examples:

1. "Design *and* implement": Both behaviors must occur.
2. "Design *or* implement": One of the two behaviors must occur.
3. "Design *and/or* implement": One or both of the two behaviors must occur.

The word "throughout" indicates that the behavior must be evident more than once (e.g., throughout the program of study). One would expect to see the behavior on several occasions (e.g., beginning, middle and end of the program) to meet the intent behind "throughout the program of study."

Strategy 4: If in doubt, refer to the rubrics. If program faculty members are unable to determine what a particular element means, they should refer to the rubrics associated with each standard and its associated elements (NASPE, 2009). The rubrics can help decipher the intent behind a particular element by describing those candidate behaviors that would indicate that a particular element has been met at the acceptable or target level of performance. In general, the rubrics can serve as another "check" to ensure that faculty members have interpreted the standards and associated elements appropriately.

If program faculty members employ those four strategies while unpacking the standards, their interpretation should align with the intent behind each standard and/or element. The ability to unpack standards is a critical variable in developing well-designed program assessments and corresponding rubrics or scoring guides that will document candidate competency.

National Initial PETE Standards & Elements Unpacked

Standard 1. Scientific and Theoretical Knowledge

Physical education teacher candidates know and apply discipline-specific scientific and theoretical concepts critical to the development of physically educated individuals.

Teacher candidates will:

1. Describe and apply physiological and biomechanical concepts related to skillful movement, physical activity and fitness.

2. Describe and apply motor learning and psychological/behavioral theory related to skillful movement, physical activity and fitness.

3. Describe and apply motor development theory and principles related to skillful movement, physical activity and fitness.

4. Identify historical, philosophical and social perspectives of physical education issues and legislation.

5. Analyze and correct critical elements of motor skills and performance concepts.

The intent behind Standard 1 is to determine the extent to which teacher candidates understand scientific and theoretical knowledge and are able to implement it in K-12 physical education instruction. Standard 1 focuses on the sub-disciplines of exercise physiology, biomechanics, motor learning, psychology and motor development, as that content and theory applies to skillful movement, physical activity and fitness. Candidates not only must demonstrate an understanding of sub-discipline content knowledge and theory, but they also must be able to implement it appropriately in the context of K-12 physical education instruction.

Candidates also must be able to identify physical education issues related to historical, philosophical and social perspectives, as well as legislation. Consequently, they must have a solid foundation in those perspectives and stay up to date on physical education legislation and related topics, such as childhood obesity.

Finally, candidates must be able to analyze and correct motor skill performance and associated "performance concepts," which are defined as:

> Knowledge and action concepts related to skillful performance of movement and fitness activities. Includes the aspects of (1) correct *selection* or "what" to do when performing a skill (e.g., when to choose a drop shot or why to choose low repetitions for strength training); and (2) correct *execution* or "how" to do a skill (e.g., executing a wrist flick or the speed of lowering the weight in a repetition). (NASPE, 2009, p. 56)

It's important to keep this definition of performance concepts in mind when designing and selecting assessments to document candidate performance specific to this element and others in which this term is indicated.

Documenting all elements within Standard 1, with the exception of Element 1.4, requires that candidates demonstrate both an understanding of the content and the ability to apply that knowledge. Consequently, program faculty members must document Standard 1 competencies with more than just a state licensure or comprehensive exam to provide sufficient evidence that candidates have met all elements within the standard.

Standard 2: Skill-Based and Fitness-Based Competence

Physical education teacher candidates are physically educated individuals with the knowledge and skills necessary to demonstrate competent movement performance and health-enhancing fitness as delineated in the NASPE K-12 Standards.

Teacher candidates will:

> 2.1. Demonstrate personal competence in motor skill performance for a variety of physical activities and movement patterns.
>
> 2.2. Achieve and maintain a health-enhancing level of fitness throughout the program.
>
> 2.3. Demonstrate performance concepts related to skillful movement in a variety of physical activities.

NASPE's Initial PETE Standard 2 requires teacher candidates to be physically educated individuals, which are defined within NASPE's six K-12 National Standards for Physical Education (NASPE, 2004). PETE candidates must have both the knowledge and the skills to demonstrate competent movement performance and health-enhancing fitness, as defined in NASPE's K-12 National Standards. All PETE Standard 2 elements are derived from that definition.

Initial PETE Element 2.3 requires a physical demonstration (functional understanding) of performance concepts. PETE candidates must demonstrate their understanding of performance concepts through actual movement performance in an authentic context.

Element 2.1 of the Initial PETE Standards requires teacher candidates to be competent in performing a variety of physical activities and fundamental movement patterns. Element 2.3 requires candidates also to demonstrate performance concepts as they relate to skillful movement in a variety of physical activities.

Based on those elements, it becomes evident that PETE programs must assess candidates' competency in skill and performance concepts in several different types of physical activity (as opposed to providing documentation only in team sports, for example). Further, candidates must demonstrate skill performance in fundamental (locomotor, non-locomotor and manipulative) movement patterns.

Finally, Element 2.2 requires that candidates attain and maintain a health-enhancing level of fitness throughout the program. Consequently, documentation will require that program faculty members assess candidates' health-related fitness more than once. Faculty members must determine what they consider to be an acceptable level of candidate performance as it applies to attaining a health-enhancing level of fitness. They also must provide documentation indicating that candidates are able to *maintain*[ital] a health-enhancing level of fitness.

In sum, it's apparent, based on Standard 2, that teacher candidates should be physically educated people and, thus, meet the same expectation that they will have for their future students.

Standard 3: Planning and Implementation

Physical education teacher education candidates plan and implement developmentally appropriate learning experiences aligned with local, state and national standards to address the diverse needs of all students.

Teacher candidates will:

3.1. Design and implement short- and long-term plans that are linked to program and instructional goals, as well as a variety of student needs.

3.2. Develop and implement appropriate (e.g., measurable, developmentally appropriate, performance-based) goals and objectives aligned with local, state and/or national standards.

3.3. Design and implement content that is aligned with lesson objectives.

3.4. Plan for and manage resources to provide active, fair and equitable learning experiences.

3.5. Plan and adapt instruction for diverse student needs, adding specific accommodations and/or modifications for student exceptionalities.

3.6. Plan and implement progressive, sequential instruction that addresses the diverse needs of all students.

3.7. Demonstrate knowledge of current technology by planning and implementing learning experiences that require students to use technology appropriately to meet lesson objectives.

Each element of Standard 3 requires candidates to plan, develop and/or design, and implement or adapt instructional content. Program faculty members must determine what type(s) of assessment(s) will provide the most compelling case for documenting that a candidate has met Standard 3.

Standard 3 focuses on planning and implementing physical education content specific to addressing the needs of all learners, which can include differences related to learning style, culture/ethnicity, skill level, gender, socioeconomic level, disabilities and body type (e.g., obese). Elements 3.1, 3.5 and 3.6, specifically, target students' varied and diverse needs.

Effective planning is critical to successful physical education instruction. Candidates must be able to design both short-term (e.g., lessons) and long-term (e.g., units of instruction) plans linked to curriculum and instructional goals (Element 3.1). Their goals and objectives for instruction also must align with local, state and/or national standards (Element 3.2).

One way for program faculty to address these planning elements is to require that teacher candidates develop their own personal lesson/unit objectives while also documenting how the performance-based objectives align with local, state and/or national standards. That's one example of how to address Element 3.2, and it can be approached in a variety of ways. Note that Element 3.2 does not require candidates to align their objectives for instruction across local, state and national levels, but alignment must occur in at least one of the levels. Further, Element 3.2 defines what constitutes "appropriate" goals and objectives as those that are measurable, developmentally appropriate and performance-based.

Element 3.3 requires PETE candidates to align course "content" with those goals and objectives, and that the instructional objectives should drive both *what* is taught and *how* it is taught. And, according to Element 3.6, the content must be designed in such a way that it demonstrates an appropriate and logical sequence or progression based on "the diverse needs of students." Planning and implementing physical education content must entail including adaptations for students with diverse needs. Further, to meet the intent behind Element 3.5, candidates must address accommodations or modifications for students with exceptionalities.

Element 3.4 requires candidates to plan for and implement appropriate resource management during physical education instruction, and those resources should provide for learning experiences that are "active, fair and equitable." That might require candidates to organize learning activities that allow for maximum practice opportunities. That can be done in numerous ways, from partner work instead of large-group activities to using small-sided games. It also means that candidates must plan for and implement an appropriate use of space and equipment, while also managing their time (e.g., lesson pacing) appropriately.

Element 3.4's requirement of providing "fair and equitable" learning experiences also might relate to methods that teacher candidates use to select teams or groups for learning tasks and/or game-oriented activities. Again, candidates may use several means for meeting fairness and equality requirements when planning for and implementing physical education instruction.

Finally, Element 3.7 requires PETE candidates to plan and implement learning activities in which students use current and appropriate technology to attain one or more lesson objectives. For example, one lesson objective might be that students are able to track the number of steps taken to complete an orienteering task as part of an adventure activity. The teacher candidate can let students use pedometers (technology) to help them meet that lesson objective.

In summary, Standard 3 represents one of the pedagogical standards. Planning for and implementing appropriate instruction is inherent across all Standard 3 elements. When doing that, PETE candidates must:

- Address the diverse needs of all students.
- Ensure that curriculum or instructional goals align with local, state and/or national objectives.
- Demonstrate that their students use technology to attain lesson objectives.
- Ensure that content is:
  - Aligned with the instructional objectives.
  - Developmentally appropriate, based on the needs of all learners.
  - Designed to provide a logical and appropriate sequence/progression of content.

Standard 4: Instructional Delivery and Management

Physical education teacher education candidates use effective communication and pedagogical skills and strategies to enhance student engagement and learning.

Teacher candidates will:

4.1. Demonstrate effective verbal and nonverbal communication skills across a variety of instruction formats.

4.2. Implement effective demonstrations, explanations and instructional cues and prompts to link physical activity concepts to appropriate learning experiences.

4.3. Provide effective instruction feedback for skill acquisition, student learning and motivation.

4.4. Recognize the changing dynamics of the environment and adjust instructional tasks based on student responses.

4.5. Use managerial rules, routines and transitions to create and maintain a safe and effective learning environment.

4.6. Implement strategies to help students demonstrate responsible personal and social behaviors in a productive learning environment.

Standard 4 focuses on delivering physical education instruction. Teacher candidates must use effective communication, and pedagogical skills and strategies that provide students with a high-quality learning experience that engages them actively within the context of the lesson. All six elements within the standard require teacher candidates to demonstrate relevant competencies in the context of providing physical education instruction to K-12 students.

One key theme embedded in every element of Standard 4 is the use of effective communication, both verbal and nonverbal. PETE candidates must communicate directions, explanations, feedback, cues and prompts, modifications of lesson content, managerial aspects of instruction and behavioral expectations for students, all within the context of instruction. Those types of communication are primarily verbal in nature, but nonverbal communication also is important. Demonstrating how to perform a task, skill or organizational format helps students understand the task at hand. Posting classroom rules and routines also can serve as a form of effective communication.

Element 4.1 requires candidates to demonstrate competency in effective communication skills across a variety of instructional formats (e.g., teaching approaches, teaching styles, instructional models). Teachers can adopt many approaches from across the spectrum of direct-versus-indirect teaching (or, teacher-centered versus learner-centered approaches). Typically, when implementing more direct instructional formats, candidates will make primary use of spoken communication; whereas, for some indirect instructional formats, written communication (non-spoken) will serve as the primary form of communication. PETE candidates will need to demonstrate both types of communication across a variety of instructional formats.

Element 4.3 requires teacher candidates to demonstrate the ability to provide effective feedback, and that should include specific, corrective instruction intended to help improve students' skill acquisition, as well as feedback that motivates students to continue working on the task at hand. Candidates also can motivate students by using positive reinforcement (general or specific), goal-setting techniques, etc.

Standard 4 also contains a management component, found in Elements 4.5 and 4.6. Element 4.5 focuses on how teacher candidates are able to create and maintain a safe and appropriate learning environment (via mechanisms such as rules, routines/protocols, transitions, etc.), while Element 4.6 — the more challenging of the two — addresses strategies that candidates use to help students demonstrate responsible personal and social behaviors.

Program faculty members must determine what constitutes "responsible personal and social behaviors," and what types of student behaviors fall into those categories. Once that's determined, program faculty members must identify appropriate strategies that teacher candidates can use to help their students exhibit such behaviors.

Finally, Element 4.4 requires PETE candidates to show that they can recognize when it's necessary to change the learning environment and, subsequently, adjust tasks based on student responses. That is known as "reflection in action" (Schön, 1983).

Standard 5: Impact on Student Learning

Physical education teacher candidates use assessments and reflection to foster student learning and inform instructional decisions.

Teacher candidates will:

> 5.1. Select or create appropriate assessments that will measure student achievement of goals and objectives.

> 5.2. Use appropriate assessments to evaluate student learning before, during and after instruction.

> 5.3. Use the reflective cycle to implement change in teacher performance, student learning and/or instructional goals and decisions.

Inherent in Standard 5 is the concept that assessment and reflection go hand in hand. PETE candidates must assess their students to determine whether they are learning or making progress toward the goal of instruction, which is student learning (Rink, 2010).

Candidates also must assess student performance to determine their own teaching effectiveness, and the reflection cycle is a critical variable in that process. Teacher candidates must gather data on student performance specific to planned learning outcomes. Next, they must analyze and interpret the data. Candidates should consider several questions after informal or formal assessment of student performance, not the least of which should be: "What can I do to inform and improve instruction?"

Reflection must also occur during instruction, and PETE candidates should consider these reflective questions while delivering lesson content:

- Are students meeting targeted learning outcomes (objectives)?
  - If so, how can I modify the given task to make it more challenging?
  - If not, how can I simplify the task to make it more appropriate?

Typically, teachers plan task modifications in advance of the lesson, but they also must reflect on the appropriateness of modifying tasks *during* instruction.

After completing the lesson, candidates will need to reflect upon how well their students performed. Based on that determination, the next step in the reflection process is for candidates to make necessary changes based on analysis and interpretation. The last step is to repeat or continue the entire reflection cycle; it should be a never-ending process, occurring before, during and after instruction.

Element 5.1 requires PETE candidates to demonstrate the ability to select appropriate assessments that document student progress toward targeted learning outcomes or objectives. Consequently, they should familiarize themselves with many types of assessments and should demonstrate competency in designing their own assessments. Assessments should align directly with student learning outcomes and should be appropriate for the student population. Further, Element 5.2 requires that candidates assess student performance before, during and after instruction. Finally, Element 5.3 requires that candidates document the reflection cycle in a way that demonstrates changes in teacher performance, student learning and/or instructional goals and decisions. Based on the intent behind Element 5.3, those changes must occur in at least one of the designated areas (teacher performance, student learning and/or instructional goals and decisions).

NASPE's *National Standards & Guidelines for Physical Education Teacher Education* defines a philosophy of assessment clearly: "Assessment must form an integral part of each lesson and must be used to guide instructional decisions and planning." (NASPE, 2009, p. 8) Program faculty members should reflect on that philosophy as they address candidates' use of assessment and reflection in the content and design of program assessments to provide support for the standard.

Standard 6: Professionalism

Physical education teacher candidates demonstrate dispositions that are essential to becoming effective professionals.

Teacher candidates will:

> 6.1. Demonstrate behaviors that are consistent with the belief that all students can become physically educated individuals.

> 6.2. Participate in activities that enhance collaboration and lead to professional growth and development.

> 6.3. Demonstrate behaviors that are consistent with the professional ethics of highly qualified teachers.

> 6.4. Communicate in ways that convey respect and sensitivity.

Standard 6 focuses on professionalism most directly as it relates to teacher candidates' dispositions and ethical behaviors. NCATE (2008) defines professional dispositions as:

> Professional attitudes, values and beliefs demonstrated through both verbal and nonverbal behaviors as educators interact with students, families, colleagues and communities. These positive behaviors support student learning and development. NCATE expects institutions to

assess professional dispositions based on observable behaviors in educational settings. The two professional dispositions that NCATE expects institutions to assess are fairness and the belief that all students can learn. (p. 89-90)

Several key aspects are embedded within that definition. First, candidate dispositions are to be based on "observable behaviors in educational settings." Candidates can demonstrate those behaviors both verbally and nonverbally through gestures, body language, etc. The dispositions should be evident as candidates interact with students, colleagues, families and community members. Finally assessment must consider the professional dispositions of "fairness" and "the belief that all students can learn," both of which are addressed in Standard 6 and Element 3.4.

Element 6.2 considers activities in which candidates choose to participate to further their professional growth and development, as well as to enhance collaboration. For example, candidates may participate in major's clubs or attend a professional workshop or state convention. Candidates can demonstrate "collaboration" when they interact with other school faculty or perhaps with parents during the student teaching/internship semester. They also could show collaboration by participating in one or more service-learning or community-based projects.

Repackaging NASPE Standards & Elements

PETE faculty members must answer two questions when determining how to go about organizing standards and elements in consideration for developing and/or selecting the six to eight assessments required for a NASPE program report. First, should NASPE elements be grouped by standard? Or, is it more logical to organize certain elements together across standards, based on the designated type of assessment? The answer to both questions is "Yes." How can that be so? For some standards and their related elements, maintaining the current organization under each standard makes sense. But certain NCATE-designated assessments (e.g., NCATE Assessment 4, Internship or Clinical Experience) are more complex and address multiple standards and elements. Consequently, an organizational format that spans standards and elements might be the best choice. Consider the following examples.

Intact Organization of Standards & Elements

For the NASPE program report, PETE programs may submit no fewer than six and up to eight assessments to document that their teacher candidates are performing at an acceptable level and to provide sufficient evidence that they are meeting all standards and elements. NCATE designates five assessments to be submitted, and PETE programs select at least one and up to three specialized professional association (SPA)-

designated assessments to submit. Program faculty members may choose to include any type of program assessment for SPA-designated assessments that helps provide evidence for meeting the standards.

For example, program faculty members might decide to develop a program assessment targeted to address Standard 2 — Skill-Based and Fitness-Based Competence — as one of the SPA-designated assessments (e.g., Assessment 6, 7 or 8) or as NCATE Assessment 2, Content Knowledge. The elements that constitute the standard can be bundled in such a manner as to provide a strong, appropriate program assessment that documents candidate performance on all associated Standard 2 elements. Program faculty can choose to pair Elements 2.1 and 2.3 together, while addressing Element 2.2 individually within a single program assessment.

Regardless of the format, PETE faculty members should group together assessment components specific to each element so that they can derive a sub-component score for each element, rather than mixing or co-mingling the elements. Providing sub-component scores for each element within a program assessment is an important guideline to follow in developing appropriate assessments and related scoring guides, because program faculty members will need to document that each element within a standard has been met.

Reorganization Across Standards & Elements

In contrast to the preceding example, in which elements within the same standard are kept intact, certain types of NCATE-designated assessments don't lend themselves to that organizational design. For example, NASPE/NCATE Assessment 4 — Internship or Clinical Experience (e.g., student teaching assessment) — is a comprehensive assessment. Most PETE faculty members would agree that this assessment addresses multiple standards and elements. One could make a case that documentation for the following elements is found within the student teaching assessment:

- All Standard 3 elements.
- All Standard 4 elements.
- Partial evidence for Elements 1.1, 1.2, 1.3 and 1.5.
- Evidence for Elements 6.1, 6.3 and 6.4.

One also could make the case that this single program assessment addresses additional elements. Regardless, it's apparent that more than one standard and its related elements are found. Program faculty members must determine which standards and elements provide the most compelling evidence specific to the assessment. If a single item on the assessment provides only a small amount of evidence for a particular element, it would be best not to include it. The same element(s) might be addressed more significantly in another program assessment.

Conclusion

We can't overemphasize the importance of accurately interpreting the intent behind the standards and elements. Precise interpretation is the key to developing and designing program assessments and scoring guides/rubrics that align clearly with the standards, and the unpacking strategies recommended in this chapter can help PETE faculty members ensure that alignment. We encourage programs to consider carefully the best way to repackage standards and elements when designing program assessments and associated scoring guides/rubrics. Assessments and rubrics that are aligned directly with the standards and elements provide an accurate depiction of program quality and candidate competency.

Chapter 6
Compiling the NCATE SPA Program Report

This chapter is directed primarily toward PETE program faculty members who will be compiling a specialized professional association (SPA) program report for national recognition. The information we share in this chapter about the program review process and about program report submission for SPA national recognition is beneficial to any teacher education program that must submit a SPA program report.

We begin with a brief overview of the SPA program report and, later, address each of its sections in detail as it applies to the NASPE SPA program report. The chapter also explores special considerations, submission options, the NASPE program review process and SPA recognition decisions. It concludes with resource options for understanding the program review process based on NCATE documentation.

NCATE SPA Program Report Overview

The NCATE SPA program report requires program faculty to provide data on six to eight comprehensive assessments that demonstrate candidate mastery of all standards and/or elements. Key questions that program reviewers consider as they examine the program report include:

1. Have candidates mastered the necessary knowledge for subjects that they will teach or jobs that they will perform?
2. Do candidates meet state licensure requirements?
3. Do candidates understand teaching and learning, and can they plan their teaching or fulfill other professional education responsibilities?
4. Can candidates apply their knowledge in classrooms and schools?
5. Do candidates focus on student learning? (NASPE, 2005)

The NCATE SPA program report is the only document that program reviewers use to judge the quality of a program and its candidates for national recognition. Therefore, it's critical for program faculty to compile the most comprehensive and compelling report, so that reviewers will respond in the affirmative to the questions listed above.

It's important to understand the SPA program report's role in relation to the institution's teacher education unit. The teacher education unit is comprised of all professional education programs (e.g., physical education, health education, math education, science education) that lead to teacher or other (e.g., librarian) school professional licensure. The program report is a SPA report, and each program within an institution's teacher education unit is affiliated with a SPA (e.g., NASPE, AAHE). Many PETE programs use NASPE's National Standards for Initial Physical Education Teacher Education as the framework for constituting the knowledge, skills and dispositions of a beginning physical education teacher, and they develop program assessments based on those standards to provide evidence of teacher candidate competency.

PETE programs submit their SPA program reports to NASPE for review. Similarly, health education teacher education programs seeking national recognition adhere to AAHE standards and submit their SPA program reports to AAHE for review. Programs that prepare candidates for dual licensure (e.g., physical education and health education) must submit separate SPA program reports to NASPE and to AAHE, if seeking national recognition in both licensure areas.

SPA reports are tied directly to an institution's teacher education unit seeking NCATE accreditation. The teacher education unit must address NCATE unit standards (similar to how licensure programs must address SPA standards and/or elements). NCATE Unit Standard 1 focuses on candidate knowledge, skills and dispositions. Each licensure program within a teacher education unit provides evidence specific to NCATE Unit Standard 1 through its SPA program report, contributing documentation of candidate performance specific to knowledge, skills and dispositions on a program-by-program basis. NCATE's Board of Examiners uses the compilation of all SPA program reports as it reviews the teacher education unit to determine whether the unit as a whole has met NCATE Unit Standard 1.

Dormant & Small Programs

In the cases of dormant programs and small programs, NCATE doesn't require a program report. Dormant programs are those in which no teacher candidates are in the pipeline and no candidate has graduated from the program within the previous three years. Programs can "reactivate" once they admit new candidates and, at that time, can choose to submit a program report.

Small programs are defined as those having five or fewer completers within the previous three years. NCATE is collaborating with states, institutions and SPAs on how these programs should be reviewed to provide quality assurance. NCATE encourages small teacher education programs to continue tracking data specific to the six to eight program assessments that it requires to oversee candidate performance. Faculty members in small programs should use a careful lens in their analysis and interpretation, as data from a small number of candidates might not provide an accurate depiction of what is actually occurring in the program or how candidates are performing. Still, trends might emerge over time.

Multiple-Level Programs

Institutions might have more than one program within the licensure area that must be reviewed for SPA national recognition. Typically, programs have an undergraduate initial licensure program but also might offer a graduate-level initial PETE program (e.g., Master of Arts in Teaching, or M.A.T.), as well. The question then becomes: "How many program reports must be submitted?" The criteria for determining the number of program reports to submit are:

- Multiple-level programs (e.g., B.S., M.A.T.) may submit linked program reports if the assessments in both program levels are identical. Every program level that needs a decision on its alignment with standards must create and submit an Accreditation Information Management System (AIMS)/Program Review Submissions (PRS) shell. In a linked report, the compiler develops the first report — typically, the undergraduate report — and then links the first report to a second report. AIMS/PRS automatically populates the second report with all the information provided in the first report. Then, the compiler can go into the second report and edit the information (e.g., change the level of the degree). Data charts for all assessments must provide disaggregated data for each linked program that reflect candidate performance for each respective program level.
- Separate program reports are required if enough differences among program levels exist in assessment structure, content and/or conceptual frameworks.

Submitting an Initial NASPE SPA Program Report

There are three types of SPA program reports: 1) initial reports, 2) Response to Conditions reports and 3) revised reports. This section explores submitting an initial NASPE SPA program report (Option A Program Report Form). Subsequent sections address writing Response to Conditions and revised program reports. Find a copy of the NASPE SPA program report in Appendix B. It might be helpful to refer to Appendix B throughout this chapter, as each section of the report is addressed.

All SPA program reports consist of a cover sheet and these major five sections:

I. Context.

II. List of Assessments.

III. Relationship of Assessments to Standards.

IV. Evidence for Meeting Standards.

V. Use of Assessment Results to Improve Program.

The cover sheet for the SPA program report consists of information specific to the report compiler, NCATE coordinator, program and institution. The required information is self-explanatory.

Section I: Context

The first section of the SPA program report pertains to context and consists of six items.

Item 1 asks for a description of any state or institutional policies that might influence the program's application of the SPA standards. It's particularly important that the report compiler describes unique state or institutional policies that might limit the program's ability to meet the SPA standards to the fullest extent. For example, some institutions might be limited in their ability to meet SPA standards due to a state-mandated credit-hour limit for undergraduate degree programs.

It's important for program faculty members to review all institutional and state-level policies that might affect the licensure program's ability to address the SPA standards and/or elements, and for the report compiler to describe those policies in this context.

Item 2 requires a description of program field and clinical experiences. The report compiler must report the number of hours for all early field experiences and the number of hours per week dedicated to student teaching or internships. Merely listing the names of the various field experiences is not sufficient; the report should include a complete description that provides an accurate picture of each field experience. For example: Is the field experience conducted in a rural, urban or suburban setting? What are the school population demographics within which these experiences occur? Do field experiences occur in diverse settings? What types of responsibilities (e.g., observation, working one on one, small-group experiences, leading warm-ups, teaching an entire class) are required of teacher candidates during various field experiences? Do candidates teach at single-site or dual-site placements (elementary, middle and/or high school) during the student teaching/internship experience?

A detailed description of the various field experience contexts provides reviewers with a more comprehensive picture of both field experiences and student teaching or internships conducted within the program.

Item 3 of Section I — Context — is an attachment that represents the program of study, outlining all courses and experiences required of candidates for degree completion. The program of study must list all course titles. Report compilers should list course prefixes, in addition to course titles, to provide program reviewers with a clear indication of course sequencing. Compilers can use a document that provides information as presented in the institution's catalog, so long as it addresses the required information. Alternatively, an advising sheet that provides program-of-study information is acceptable. It's also permissible to scan the document and submit it in PDF format.

Item 4 of the context is where the report compiler can attach any tables or graphics that pertain to Items 1 and 2, since the PRS system does not allow tables or graphics to be embedded within those text fields. Be sure that the file title is representative of the content.

Item 5 addresses candidate information. Report compilers must provide three years' worth of data on candidates currently enrolled in the program and on those who have completed the program, starting with the most recent academic year. NCATE uses the Title II definition of "program completer," which one can find in the online SPA program report (or refer to Appendix B). Data are to be reported separately for each program level and for programs offered at more than one site.

Item 6 pertains to faculty information. The Faculty Information chart consists of information about program faculty members responsible for professional coursework, clinical supervision and those who teach program methods courses. Report compilers import faculty information from the NCATE coordinator's faculty information chart in the AIMS/PRS system. The report lists up to three contributions over the previous three years for each faculty member in the categories of scholarship, leadership in professional associations and service.

Section II: List of Assessments

Similar to the program report cover sheet page of the SPA program report, Section II of the SPA program report takes minimal time to complete. The report compiler lists the names of each of the six to eight program assessments submitted as evidence for meeting the SPA standards. The type or form of each program assessment (e.g., exam, lesson plan, unit plan, movement skills test, fitness test, case study, project, reflection) also must be indicated, along with identification of when the assessment is administered within the licensure program.

Required Assessments for SPA Program Reports

NCATE identifies the "type or form" of assessments required for Assessments 1-5 in the SPA program report. Assessment 6 also is required, but NCATE doesn't prescribe the type or form of assessment to be used. For Assessment 6, program faculty members select an assessment of their own choosing that helps to document that all NASPE standards and elements have been met. Assessments 7 and 8 are optional assessments that programs can use to document sufficient evidence that all standards and elements are met.

Assessment 1: Licensure assessment, or other content-based assessment.
Assessment 1 requires scores from the content knowledge state licensure test. Many states require program graduates to complete one or more of the Praxis Series™ tests, but some states have developed their own content-knowledge licensure exams. The report compiler is expected to show the alignment of the state licensure exam content with SPA Standards. NCATE policy requires that program candidates attain at least an 80 percent pass rate on the designated state licensure content-knowledge exam for the program *in the most recent year* to qualify for national SPA recognition. NCATE requirements for the state licensure test data are outlined here:

- Licensure test data must reflect the percentage of teacher candidates who passed the state licensure test in the most recent year. Providing data from three years, NCATE says, is "optimal."
- The most recent year of data should include total scores and, if possible, sub-scores on the licensure test.
- The data summary table must include the state cut (passing) score.
- Data must be presented for all program completers, even if fewer than 10 graduates take the exam within the given year.

For programs within a state that doesn't require a content-knowledge state licensure exam, report compilers must include data from another assessment to document candidates' attainment of content knowledge for Assessment 1.

Assessment 2: Content knowledge in physical education. Assessment 2 also must address content knowledge, but program faculty members select the type of assessment to use. Assessment 2 is a logical place to address Elements 2.1, 2.2 and 2.3 under NASPE Standard 2, which requires documentation of teacher candidate ability to demonstrate competent movement performance and health-enhancing fitness. Comprehensive exams, health-related fitness assessments, fundamental movement skills assessments, and assessments of performance-competency and game play are some examples of assessments that programs could include for Assessment 2.

Alternatively, some program faculty members might want to consider using course grades to demonstrate candidate competency in physical education content knowledge, although we don't recommend that option. Based on NCATE directives, all SPAs will accept course grades as one of the six to eight key assessments submitted in the program report. Programs that choose to use course grades as a program assessment must follow detailed guidelines and formatting requirements. Refer to Appendix A or visit www.ncate.org/Accreditation/ProgramReview/GuidelinesandProcedures/Documenting CourseGrades/tabid/456/Default.aspx.

Assessment 3: Candidate ability to plan instruction. Assessment 3 must document teacher candidates' ability to plan effectively and implement developmentally appropriate learning experiences. Typically, assessments specific to lesson or unit plans (or other program planning assessments, such as individualized education plans, needs assessments or intervention plans) are used to meet the intent of this assessment. Programs choose the type of planning and implementation to be documented.

Assessment 4: Internship or clinical experiences. Assessment 4 must be an observation instrument demonstrating that candidates' knowledge, skills and dispositions are implemented effectively. Programs should use the assessment used during the student teaching/internship experience for Assessment 4. Many departments have developed their own student teaching observation instruments to use, while other institutions require all teacher licensure programs to assess student teachers using the same assessment instrument.

Assessment 5: Candidate effect on student learning. Assessment 5 must document candidates' ability to affect student learning. While candidates can satisfy that requirement by demonstrating their ability to implement assessments, they also must demonstrate their ability to use information gathered through K-12 assessment and reflect on changes in teaching and/or instruction to adjust future lessons. Assessment 5 is more than a set of assessments; candidates must document that their teaching affected student learning. Also, learning must have occurred over time, so the period between pre- and post-assessment must be sufficient to support student learning. Student work samples, IEPs, case studies and implemented unit plans are examples of assessments that programs might use to fulfill Assessment 5.

Guidelines for Selecting NASPE SPA Program Assessments

PETE program faculty members should consider the following guidelines specific to Section II of the program report when determining which program assessments to include in the NASPE SPA program report.

1. Select the most compelling and comprehensive assessments that, when reviewed, provide sufficient evidence that teacher candidates meet SPA standards. NASPE requires initial PETE programs to meet all elements listed under each standard (NASPE, 2009) before granting NASPE national recognition. When selecting assessments for a NASPE program report using the 2008 standards, program faculty members should choose broad assessments that have the potential to address several standards/elements. Programs have only eight assessments with which to demonstrate teacher candidate competence, so each program assessment selected for a NASPE SPA program report should address multiple NASPE elements. Although that might seem daunting, it can be accomplished with preplanning.

2. Each selected program assessment must be administered to all teacher candidates.

3. Generic assessments, such as those used by the teacher education unit (e.g., student teaching assessments), usually are not aligned directly with NASPE Standards. Therefore, PETE faculty members might wish to include a bridge rubric (see Chapter 3) or an addendum. A bridge rubric can address specific SPA standards that are not addressed clearly in the unit assessment.

Appendix C provides a template for program faculty to identify assessments for each element of NASPE's Initial PETE Standards.

Section III: Relationship of Assessments to Standards

Section III of the SPA program report serves a dual purpose. First, it indicates to the program whether at least one assessment addresses each element to provide evidence that the standard has been met. Second, Section III serves as a roadmap for program reviewers. It indicates which assessments reviewers should consider for evidence of meeting a specific element and/or standard. PETE faculty members must determine which assessments provide the most compelling evidence for a particular element or standard, rather than identifying every assessment for every standard and/or element. If compilers identify all assessments for each standard, it can indicate to program reviewers one of three possibilities:

1. Program faculty members didn't carefully select assessments critical to providing evidence specific to the element.

2. Program faculty didn't have enough evidence — or didn't have confidence in their evidence — and, therefore, chose to list all assessments in hopes that reviewers might find enough evidence that the standard had been met.

3. Program faculty didn't understand the intent of the standard and/or element fully.

Generally, no more than three assessments should be necessary to provide enough evidence that an element/standard has been met. If that's not the case, program faculty members should re-examine the assessments to determine whether they provide the evidence needed to demonstrate that the standards and elements have been met.

To complete Section III, report compilers must complete the chart provided in the SPA program report AIMS/PRS shell. Section III identifies program assessments for each of the 28 initial PETE elements.

Section IV: Evidence for Meeting Standards

Section IV is the heart of the program report; this is where report compilers make the most compelling case that the program has met each of the standards and elements. Documentation for each program assessment consists of two major components: (1) a narrative section and (2) assessment documentation. Report compilers must address both components for each listed program assessment. They should create a single file for each assessment that includes the narrative section and the assessment documentation, and should use this naming methodology for each assessment file: Assessment number – Name of specific assessment (e.g., Assessment 3 – Unit Plan, Assessment 4 – Student Teaching/Internship Assessment, etc.).

Narrative Section. The narrative section for each assessment in Section IV may be up to two pages long and must address these four items (NCATE, 2011a):

1. A brief description of the assessment and its use in the program.
2. A description of how this assessment aligns with SPA standards and elements, as cited in Section III, Relationships of Assessments to Standards. (Cite SPA standards and elements by number: Element 3 of Standard 2 should be cited as 2.3.)
3. A brief analysis of the data findings.
4. An interpretation of how the data provide convincing evidence for meeting the identified SPA standards and elements. (Again, cite by number as in Item 2 above.)

Within the Section IV narrative component, report compilers must provide a brief description of the assessment and its use within the program (Item 1 above). Second, they must provide a description of how the assessment aligns with the SPA standards and elements (Item 2 above). One way to convey the response to Item 2 is by creating an assessment/standards (or elements) alignment table. Figure 6.1 represents a partial example specific to NCATE Assessment 3, in which program faculty members selected a lesson plan to serve as the required planning assessment.

Figure 6.1. Alignment of Assessment Components With NASPE Elements

Assessment Component	Aligns w/NASPE Element(s)
Lesson Objectives	Elements 3.1 & 3.2
Content Development	Elements 3.3, 3.5 & 3.6
Accommodations or Adaptations	Element 3.5
Management Aspects	Element 3.4

Report compilers also might include sub-components under the various assessment components included within the alignment table. The more detailed the table, the easier it will be for program reviewers to determine the alignment. Each assessment component indicated in the alignment table should align directly with the identified standards and/or elements. It's not required that program faculty members create a table to demonstrate alignment, but it can provide a succinct means of presenting the necessary information.

Item 3 of the narrative requires a brief analysis of candidate data for the designated program assessment. The report of data analysis for each assessment in Section IV should be short and concise and should address these questions:

- What did the general findings indicate based on candidate performance?
- Are candidates performing at an acceptable level? (Make sure that the "acceptable" level is clear to reviewers.)

Finally, Item 4 requires program compilers to interpret assessment data and make a case that SPA standards and elements identified in Item 2 have been met. Report compilers should take into consideration the strength of the evidence and present the case on an individual basis for each assessment.

Assessment Documentation. This is the second major component addressed for each assessment as reported in Section IV of the program report. The assessment documentation consists of three items:

1. The assessment tool itself, or the actual assignment (e.g., project) handout provided to teacher candidates.
2. The scoring guide for the assessment/assignment.
3. Candidate data derived from the assessment (data summary table).

Assessment Tool/Assignment. Report compilers must include the assessment tool/instrument or actual detailed assignment or project, as provided to teacher candidates (except for the state licensure exam). The actual assignment or project (if applicable) given to candidates provides reviewers with a clear understanding of the assessment requirements. If the assessment is course-embedded (e.g., unit plan), for example, report compilers should include the entire unit plan assignment.

Scoring Guide. Next, report compilers should provide the scoring guide for the assessment/assignment, along with each component, category and/or sub-category of the assessment tool/assignment, exactly as it appears in the assessment/assignment. The purpose of the scoring guide is to indicate levels of candidate performance, as developed by the program. A minimum of two levels ("acceptable" and "unacceptable") is required, but most programs include a "target" level of performance, as well, to indicate the preferred level of teacher candidate performance. See Chapter 3 for a description of how to write rubrics for program assessments.

Since most, if not all, of the assessments chosen for the program report are used to satisfy multiple standards (and elements), report compilers must show scores for each sub-category of the assessment to document candidate performance specific to particular standards and elements. That's why, in Chapter 3, we suggested using analytic rubrics so that the sub-categories of an assessment are readily apparent. A total cumulative score on an assessment as found on a holistic rubric doesn't give reviewers enough information to determine whether designated standards/elements have been met.

When preparing the program report, compilers must state which level of performance is "acceptable" if the rubric or scoring guide doesn't use that term. Also, report compilers should examine the level of rigor for an acceptable performance. The criteria for "acceptable" must meet the intent of the standard or element that the assessment addresses. Reviewers shouldn't have to question whether candidates actually performed at an acceptable level for the various standards or elements.

Data Summary Table. This is the last item of documentation included for each designated assessment. The data summary table for each assessment must provide assessment data from two applications for an initial program report submission. For example, if an assessment is course-embedded, and the course is offered during both fall and spring semesters, this would constitute two applications of assessment data. If the course is offered only once a year, however, it would take two years to acquire data from two applications of the assessment. When developing the data summary table, report compilers should label candidate data by semester and year, or year (if the assessment is administered only once a year) and indicate the percentage of candidates achieving at each level of performance (e.g., unacceptable, acceptable, target).

The most recent application of assessment data should be presented first, followed by previous data applications. The data table must indicate clearly the minimal acceptable level of candidate performance for the designated assessment. Report compilers can use an asterisk or other symbol to indicate the minimal acceptable level of performance in the data summary table and include a simple explanation directly below the data table (e.g., * = minimal acceptable level of candidate performance).

When designing the assessment, scoring guide and associated data summary table, it's important to show the direct alignment of SPA standards and elements on all three documents to provide a clear and succinct connection. That will save reviewers from having to spend time determining which standards or elements the assessment addresses. Refer to Appendix D, NCATE Assessment 3: Lesson Plan, for an example.

Reviewers' Perspective. Program reviewers consider Section IV to be the heart of the program report and, as such, might ask many questions as they examine it. Once the report compiler has completed Section IV, program faculty members should double-check the content by determining whether they can respond "Yes" to each of the following questions, as adapted from Martin and Judd (2006):

1. Do the assessments align with SPA standards (and/or elements)?
2. Do the assessments discern meaningful cognitive demands and skill requirements at challenging levels for candidates?
3. Are assessments accurate and free from bias?
4. Do scoring guides/rubrics provide clear and distinct levels of candidate performance and is the "acceptable" level defined clearly?
5. Do scoring guides/rubrics address all components on the assessment tool or assignment?

6. Does the minimal level of candidate performance, as determined by the program, meet the intent of the standards/elements with which it is aligned?

7. Do the data, as reported, indicate the extent to which candidates meet the standards/ elements?

8. Have the standards/elements been met?

Those questions serve as a good gauge for program faculty members to determine how well they've addressed the task of designing and implementing assessment tools/ assignments and associated scoring guides and to ensure that the data summary tables reflect candidate competency.

Section V: Use of Assessment Results to Improve the Program

This is the last section of the program report for those submitting an initial program report. It's also perhaps the most important section for the program's future, because it relates to self-study and program evaluation. The purpose of Section V is two-fold:

1. To document that the program has analyzed and interpreted candidate assessment data specific to the quality of both teacher candidates and the teacher licensure program.

2. To document that evidence of proposed or incorporated programmatic changes is addressed, based on interpretation of the data.

For Section V, report compilers must write a narrative to describe the analysis, interpretation and proposed changes derived from examining teacher candidate data using the framework of NCATE Unit Standard 1: (a) content knowledge; (b) pedagogical and professional knowledge, skills and dispositions; and (c) effects on P-12 student learning. This means that report compilers must write a separate narrative section specific to each of the content areas of NCATE Unit Standard 1 (listed below). Principal data findings for each content area should be synthesized, rather than presented in an assessment-by-assessment format.

1. *Content knowledge.* In this narrative, report compilers consider data gathered from Assessments 1 and 2, which address content knowledge, along with program faculty members' input specific to the analysis and interpretation conducted. Compilers also should describe program changes made or proposed as a result of examining the data specific to content knowledge.

2. *Pedagogical and professional knowledge, skills and dispositions.* Assessments 3 and 4 provide evidence for this section of the narrative.

3. *Student learning.* Assessment 5 provides direct evidence of student learning and may serve as a major discussion point as addressed in this narrative.

Report compilers also must determine the focus of Assessment 6, which is required. If Assessments 7 and/or 8 are included in the program report, the compiler also must determine the focus of these assessments relative to Unit Standard 1 content within the Section V narratives, because they are considered optional assessments.

Report compilers should follow this advice on preparing each narrative:

1. Summarize principal findings from the evidence (appropriate assessment data).
2. Provide the program's interpretation of the findings.
3. Describe programmatic or curricular changes made or proposed based on faculty members' interpretation and recommendations.
4. Describe steps that the program has taken to use data from the assessments for improving candidate and program quality.

Section V concludes the program report content required for an initial SPA program report.

The SPA program report template provides all guidelines for attachments and formatting for all types of program reports (initial, revised and Response to Conditions reports). We chose not to discuss these guidelines here because parameters could easily change at any time.

The NASPE Program Review Process

This section explores the SPA program review process for NASPE, as outlined here:

1. Once report compilers submit the program report in the AIMS/PRS system, the review process begins. NCATE first checks to ensure that submission and formatting guidelines are met.
2. The NASPE SPA liaison assigns review teams of one lead reviewer and, usually, two other program reviewers to review the program report.
3. Each reviewer reviews the program report independently.
4. Members of the review team share reviews with one another and confer until they reach consensus.
5. The lead reviewer writes a team recognition report that synthesizes the review team's comments and provides a recommendation for the recognition decision.
6. A NASPE committee audits the team report and provides a national recognition decision.
7. NCATE reviews the NASPE committee's audit of the National Recognition Report and makes copy edits. If any discrepancies or areas of confusion are found, the NCATE staff reader calls it to the attention of the SPA liaison and clarifications are made.
8. NCATE notifies the program that the recognition decision is available on the AIMS/PRS system.

NCATE/SPA Recognition Decisions

NCATE/SPA recognition decisions have changed over the past several years. New guidelines for recognition decisions (NCATE, 2011b) are based on which category a program falls under: (a) not recognized previously, or (b) is recognized currently. Within each category, reviewers make one of three determinations.

For programs not recognized previously, the determinations are:

1. **National recognition contingent upon unit accreditation.** Reviewers make this determination if the program meets the standards and — for NASPE recognition — all of the elements. No further submission is required, and the program receives full national recognition when the teacher education unit receives NCATE accreditation. Or, if the teacher education unit is already accredited, the program is listed as nationally recognized.

2. **National recognition with conditions contingent upon unit accreditation.** In this case, the program generally meets the standards and associated elements, but must submit a Response to Conditions report within 18 months to address the conditions cited. Possible conditions include:

   - Insufficient data to determine whether standards/elements have been met.
   - Insufficient alignment among standards/elements, or assessments or scoring guides.
   - Lack of quality in some assessments or scoring guides.
   - An insufficient number of SPA standards have been met.
   - The NCATE requirement for an 80 percent pass rate on state licensure tests has not been met.

   NCATE provides two opportunities to remove the conditions within an 18-month period. If the conditions are met, the program then becomes nationally recognized. If, after two attempts, the program is unsuccessful, the determination is changed to "not nationally recognized."

3. **Further development required.** This determination is justified when the program has met only a few standards, or the standards that the program has not met are too critical to program quality to ignore. In this case, recognition is not appropriate. Programs that receive this designation have two opportunities within 12 to 14 months after the initial decision to attain either "national recognition" or "national recognition with conditions" designation. If unsuccessful after two attempts, the program's status will change to "not nationally recognized."

For program recognized currently, program reviewers make one of these three determinations:

1. **National recognition.** Reviewers reach this determination when a program report provides enough evidence that the program meets all SPA standards (and in NASPE's case, all elements) and documents a state licensure exam pass rate of at least 80 percent. No further documentation is required, and the program is listed as "nationally recognized."

2. **National recognition, with conditions.** The same descriptive criteria outlined in the "national recognition, with conditions" determination for programs not recognized previously apply with following exception:

> The program is listed on the NCATE Web site as "nationally recognized (based on its prior review)" until the Unit Accreditation Board makes an accreditation decision for the unit. At that point, if the program is still considered "nationally recognized, with conditions," NCATE will <u>change</u> the designation on its Web site to "national recognition, with conditions." This designation will stand until the program achieves "national recognition" status, or its status is changed to "not nationally recognized," in which case the program will be removed from the list on NCATE's Web site (NCATE, 2011b).

3. **National recognition, with probation.** This designation is appropriate if the program report did not provide sufficient evidence for meeting several SPA standards or if the standards and elements not met are critical to program quality. This indicates that the program does not warrant national recognition at this time. To remove the probation status, program faculty members can submit a new or revised program report to address unmet standards. NCATE provides two opportunities within 12 to 14 months after its initial decision to attain "national recognition" or "national recognition, with conditions" status. If a program is unsuccessful in its two attempts, its status reverts to "not nationally recognized."

For Revised and Response to Conditions Reports Only

Revised or Response to Conditions reports are submitted in the same way as initial program reports. The institution must notify NCATE via e-mail (ncateprograms@ncate.org) no later than one month before the submission deadline of the program's intention to submit a revised or Response to Conditions report. NCATE staff members will prepare a program report shell (AIMS/PRS) for this purpose once they receive notification. One application of assessment data is required for each revised or modified assessment and/or scoring guide submitted.

Submitting a Revised Program Report

Revised reports are required for programs that received a SPA recognition decision of "Further development required" or "Recognized with probation." It's not necessary to complete all sections of the program report shell as part of the revised report; reviewers have access to previous program reports via the AIMS/PRS system. Compilers and program faculty should read all comments made in the SPA report and decide how best to respond. Whether the report compiler needs to submit specific sections depends on the concerns that program reviewers raised.

Typically, revised reports document how the program now meets the NASPE standards/elements not met in the first report. At a minimum, report compilers must complete the cover sheet, indicating that this is a revised program report, complete Section VI, and submit specific responses (e.g., items in Section IV and/or Section V) and documents (e.g., assessments, scoring guides, data tables) that have changed since the original (or previous) submission, focusing particular attention on Part B: Status of Meeting SPA Standards (comments for standards/elements not met).

When program faculty members receive the SPA recognition decision, it's in the program's best interest to consider and plan the next steps in the program evaluation process immediately. Some questions to consider when working through the next steps:

- What must we address?
- What concerns or issues did the reviewers cite?
- What components must we revise or change?
- If we must revise assessments, scoring guides and data tables, who will be responsible?
- What other factors can we glean from the recognition report that will help us improve candidate competencies relative to the standards and/or elements, as well as improving overall program quality?

After making necessary changes (e.g., revising rubrics, developing assessments that align with the intent behind the element(s), data collection with revised assessments and rubrics), report compilers then complete the revised program report, beginning with the cover sheet, and then address Section VI on the AIMS/PRS system. Section VI provides the roadmap for those who will review the revised program report. Report compilers should:

1. Describe *in Section VI* what changes or additions have been made to address the standards *not met* in the original submission.
2. Provide new responses to questions and/or new documents reflecting the changes/additions *in the corresponding sections of the program report* to verify the changes described in Section VI.

Compilers also must submit appropriate documentation for Sections I, II, III, IV and/or V, as necessary, to reflect changes, additions and/or revisions made since submitting the initial program report.

Submitting a Response to Conditions Program Report

Response to Conditions reports are required for programs that receive a SPA recognition designation of "nationally recognized, with conditions." As with a revised report, report compilers need not complete all sections of the program report; reviewers can access previous reports via the AIMS/PRS system.

Report compilers submit only specific responses and documents that demonstrate changes or additions to items listed in Part G of the original recognition report. Part G outlines the conditions that the program must meet to attain national recognition. If, in the opinions of program reviewers, all conditions listed in Part G are satisfied, they will deem the program "nationally recognized."

The next steps in the program evaluation process become evident in Part G, in which program faculty members devise a plan for meeting the conditions that NASPE has stipulated in its recognition report. Often, next steps will require a revision of assessments, scoring guides and associated data tables and/or collection of new data based on revisions made. NCATE requires at least one administration or application of an assessment once revised or changed in some way, to provide data regarding candidate competency in that area.

Once PETE program faculty members have identified all necessary changes, they should create a timeline with NCATE deadlines for resubmitting the report. Typically, NCATE allows programs to resubmit twice within an 18-month period.

As soon as program revisions — as outlined under the conditions — have been made and one application of corresponding data are available, report compilers can begin to complete the Response to Conditions program report. The report compiler should enter the AIMS/PRS system and first complete the cover sheet, indicating that this is a Response to Conditions report. Next, the report compiler addresses Section VI of the report, following these instructions:

1. List all conditions found in Part G of the NASPE SPA recognition report.
2. For each condition, provide a brief narrative outlining how faculty members addressed the item.
3. Attach or insert appropriate documentation into Sections I, II, III, and/or IV, reflecting the changes/additions made in response to the conditions listed in Part G.

Submission Options for SPA Program Reports

Four submission options are available for SPA program review selection (NCATE, 2011c). Any program may choose Option A, B or D. If a program meets the criteria listed for Option C, program faculty members may choose that option or any of the other options.

Option A. This reflects the current (effective since 2004) NCATE program report submission process, with some changes to the required documentation. The program report sections discussed earlier in this chapter reflect Option A. Program faculty members select six to eight key assessments, including the five designated types of NCATE assessments, to document that all SPA standards have been met.

Option B. Although similar to Option A, Option B provides further flexibility in program assessment choice and types of assessments submitted. For Option B, program faculty members select key assessments that provide the evidence necessary for documenting that the program has met all SPA standards without having to meet all NCATE assessment types (two content knowledge assessments, planning assessment, field experience assessment and impact-on-student-learning assessment) designated in Option A. Programs that choose Option B must adhere to these guidelines:

1. Faculty members may select up to eight assessments, with no minimum number of assessments required.
2. One of the assessments submitted must be the state licensure test if a state licensure test exists in the discipline area.
3. One of the assessments submitted must focus on candidate impact on student learning, or — for non-teaching programs — an assessment of candidate impact on providing a supportive learning environment.
4. Assessments, taken as a whole, must demonstrate mastery of SPA standards.
5. Assessments must address the following key elements of NCATE Unit Standard 1: content, pedagogical content knowledge and skills, and impact on student learning (NCATE, 2010c).

Option C. This option is available to programs deemed "nationally recognized" using the Option A six- to eight-key assessment model on their previous review cycle and are submitting to SPAs whose standards have not changed since the most recent submission of their program report. The amount of information required for program report submission is significantly less in Option C than for Option A, although these aspects must be addressed:

1. Data must be submitted on all assessments.
2. Documentation must be submitted only for those assessments that are new or changed substantially since the previous submission.
3. Section I must be completed only for items in which there has been substantial change since the previous submission.
4. Section V should focus on how the program has used data to improve.

Option D, *Validity and Reliability Studies*. NCATE describes this option thus:

> This option permits an institution to conduct validity and reliability studies of its assessments in lieu of other program report evidence requirements. The validity and reliability of assessments (content in relation to standards, consistency with other evidence, success in subsequent employment, etc.) is so integral to a standards- and performance-based national recognition review that systematic examination of validity is essential. It would, by definition, directly address SPA standards. It would permit institutions with appropriately prepared faculty to formulate a task as part of accreditation that is meaningful for them, while, not unimportantly, helping to advance the research base for educator preparation. It is an

option that might lend itself to joint participation across several institutions, or at least across programs within an institution. It is probably not an option that every institution has the capacity to execute; moreover, it would require a different kind of selection and/or training of reviewers. Before a program could choose this option, it must receive approval from NCATE. (NCATE, 2011c)

In sum, program faculty members do have a choice of submission options for SPA program reports. They can choose to continue to submit under the current process (Option A), but they also should consider determining which option provides the best opportunity to make the most compelling case that the program has met the SPA standards. We recommend that, because most submission options are fairly new, program faculty members seek input from NCATE when considering a different submission option.

NCATE Resources for Submitting Program Reports

NCATE's program review process continues to evolve and be refined. As such, it's important for program faculty members to stay current by using the resources available on NCATE's Web sites. The following resources are available at www.ncate.org/Accreditation/ProgramReview/GuidelinesandProcedures/tabid/441/Default.aspx.

- Guidelines on Programs to Be Submitted.
- Guidelines on Data.
- Program Report Submission Due Dates and Timelines.
- Guidelines on Assessment.
- Guidelines on Decisions.
- New Options for Program Review.
- Guidelines for Submitting Initial Licensure/Post-Baccalaureate (IL/PB) Program Reports.
- Guidelines for Submitting Option C Program Reports.
- Documenting Course Grades.
- SPA Assessment Library.

The following resources are available from the Program Review NCATE Web site found at: http://www.ncate.org/Accreditation/ProgramReview/tabid/116/Default.aspx.

- Program Review Process.
- Guidelines and Procedures.
- Program Report Submission.
- Praxis II Data for NCATE Standard One.

- Program Review System FAQ.
- Program Review System (PRS) Help.
- Program Review Resources.

We strongly encourage program faculty members to check NCATE's Web sites often for updated and current information on the program review process.

Conclusion

Writing a SPA program report for national recognition is a comprehensive, detail-oriented endeavor, with specific guidelines and requirements. The goal for program faculty members should be to provide clear and convincing evidence that candidates perform at an acceptable level when held to a designated set of standards. Programs that buy into continuous program evaluation will find that writing a program report for accreditation purposes becomes relatively manageable.

Chapter 7

Working Through the Process

In this chapter, we address the process and strategies related to conducting a proper program evaluation for any academic program, including an evaluation intended for submission as an accreditation or national recognition report. We begin by explaining how to develop a plan for program evaluation, then explore management and organization-related aspects such as roles and responsibilities, assessment implementation plans and monitoring, candidate artifacts, establishing timelines, etc. Finally, we offer an example of a program/curriculum review and redesign to provide readers with an authentic representation of how program faculty members can work through the process.

Developing a Plan for Program Evaluation

Academic programs that aim to begin a system of continuous program review/evaluation for accreditation or national recognition , departmental purposes, unit evaluations, program improvement or other related initiatives should follow the eight-step process described in Chapter 1. First, consider what program faculty members know (or want to know) about the program's quality and the competencies of its candidates (Step 1). What framework will program faculty members use to determine candidate competencies specific to the program? Many academic programs will choose to evaluate the program based on state and/or national standards, but they also can develop criteria on which to judge the quality of program candidates.

Whether program faculty members develop separate criteria or use standards to provide a framework for comparison, they will need to determine where the criteria or standards are addressed within the program of study. If the program has submitted reports for accreditation or national recognition previously, program faculty members can use those results and feedback to determine the questions they wish to consider in Step 1. Once the questions, standards or program criteria are determined, program faculty members can initiate a systematic plan of action.

How are candidates assessed relative to the program's selected criteria? Are gaps evident in addressing the standards or selected criteria? Program faculty members must select and/or develop program assessments that will provide evidence of candidate competency specific to the selected program criteria (Step 2). Then, they must gather assessment data over time (Step 3) and analyze those data for trends. Interpreting the findings or results occurs during the subsequent program evaluation process (Step 4), resulting in the rendering of judgments of program quality (Step 5).

Next, program faculty members must make explicit and informed decisions regarding program and curriculum changes to improve program and candidate quality (Step 6). They then implement the changes (Step 7). Ultimately, this cyclical process of program evaluation continues (Step 8). It is never ending, and the goal is to always strive for improved program quality and candidate competency.

Management- and Organization-Related Aspects of Program Evaluation

The task of conducting a quality program evaluation might seem daunting, but if program faculty members address the management- and organization-related aspects of program evaluation early on, the task will be manageable. Determining how to tackle those aspects in advance will lessen the uneasiness and discomfort so often associated with the program evaluation process.

The Program Coordinator

One of the most critical decisions in the program evaluation process is selecting a program coordinator to oversee and administer the process. The person selected must have comprehensive knowledge of the academic program and the program evaluation process. More important, he or she must possess excellent organization, management and leadership skills. The program coordinator must be able to delegate roles and responsibilities to other faculty members, set deadlines and ensure that the work is completed. This person should be experienced and must have his or her colleagues' trust, to ensure that a productive experience occurs.

The program coordinator should be a senior, tenured faculty member (Senne, 2006). It would be counterproductive to select a junior, non-tenured faculty member for this role, no matter how knowledgeable in program evaluation/accreditation processes the person might be. The task of coordinating a program review is intensely time-consuming and, unless a dedicated and substantial amount of release time is provided, the program will run the risk of limited scholarship. As a general guideline, junior faculty members should be assigned less demanding roles in the program evaluation process.

Faculty Buy-In & Decision-Making

Faculty buy-in is of utmost importance in conducting an effective program evaluation. All program faculty members must buy into the notion that continuous, systematic program evaluation is essential for a program to improve in quality. Continuous program improvement will ensure candidate competency and reflect appropriate changes based on current education, health and physical activity trends, and state and national standards to meet the needs of the targeted population. Thoughtful and deliberate dialogue must occur to reach consensus on program and curriculum decisions. Strong leadership from the program coordinator and dedication from the faculty provide a formula for success in this endeavor.

Faculty Roles & Responsibilities

The program evaluation process should be a team endeavor, with each faculty member contributing to the end product — program evaluation — by assuming various roles and responsibilities. The program coordinator should devote much thought to matching program evaluation tasks with individual faculty members. Ensuring that program evaluation roles and responsibilities are manageable for each faculty member is, in part, the key to success. What special expertise and talents are available, and how would those best be matched with the tasks at hand?

Delegating program evaluation responsibilities appropriately, based on individual faculty members' strengths, will yield a better overall product. The program coordinator should begin this process by generating a list of all responsibilities and/or tasks that must be completed during the program review. After the list is generated, the program coordinator can begin to match tasks and responsibilities with program faculty members, based on expertise, strengths and time availability. Subsequently, the program coordinator should meet with each faculty member individually to discuss proposed program evaluation assignments. To secure support from each faculty member for the program evaluation, it's important to provide a strong rationale for the tasks assigned. Securing that buy-in in advance will alleviate many problems down the road and will provide a clear set of expectations for all.

The Report Compiler

The information in this section is relevant to submitting program reports for external review (e.g., NASPE national recognition). It might not be necessary to appoint a report compiler if the report is simply for internal review and self-improvement.

The report compiler is charged with clearly and accurately conveying program faculty members' response — based on consensus — on each aspect of the program to be addressed within the report. The report compiler shouldn't be the sole person developing responses for each section of the program report; rather, he or she must serve as the conduit for communicating faculty consensus regarding each section of the program report. For that reason, the report compiler must have strong technical writing skills and the ability to communicate accurately what the program and its candidates are accomplishing. That information is what program reviewers will use to render their decision regarding program quality and candidate competency, so it must be accurate, clear and compelling.

It's imperative that the report compiler begin writing sections of the program report as soon as information is accessible. Once data are available from the first application of a particular assessment, for example, the compiler can create a data summary table. After the same assessment is administered a second time, those data should be entered. It makes sense to write the various report sections as program faculty members complete the necessary tasks associated with each section. Waiting until all information is available can lead to rushing to complete the report on time.

Finally, it will be worthwhile for the program coordinator to review each section of the compiler's draft report carefully, to ensure that information is communicated accurately and appropriately. The program coordinator should assume full responsibility for the report's content. Reviewing each section as the report compiler completes it will allow time for necessary changes, edits and revisions prior to submission. If the program coordinator is also the report compiler, another knowledgeable colleague should read the report section drafts as they're completed.

Assessment Implementation Plans and Monitoring

Once the assessments to be used in the program review are selected, faculty members must determine how and when they will be administered. Some program assessments are likely to be course-embedded. In that case, the assessments will be administered during the semester(s) in which the courses are offered. Typically, an assessment such as a student teaching evaluation or internship evaluation will occur toward the end of the student teaching or internship experience. In contrast, assessments such as candidate dispositions might be conducted on a systematic basis at various points throughout a program, resulting in more than one test administration during a candidate's program of study. In such cases, it will be necessary to determine when these types of assessments will occur. For example, program faculty members might choose to conduct a candidate dispositions assessment first during initial entry-level courses, again during the teaching methods course and again during student teaching.

Program faculty members also might elect to create decision points to provide gateways to the next series of courses in the program of study. In that case, the first decision point might occur after students complete the basic core of general education courses, when program faculty members review candidates' cumulative GPA to ensure that they have completed all required general education courses. A second decision point might occur after preliminary coursework in a major, just before starting teaching methods courses or at the start of intensive lab-based courses or field-based practica. A third decision point might occur before the final field placement, when faculty members determine whether candidates have the skills necessary to succeed in the workplace. At the final decision point, program faculty members would consider candidates' readiness to graduate from the program and would use results from the internship/student teaching placement and scores on the final content exam (e.g., Praxis™ II, ACSM comprehensive exam) to determine whether candidates have the skills, knowledge, abilities and dispositions to earn a degree.

One advantage to creating decision points is that it allows program faculty members to screen out candidates who are not doing well before they progress too far to change their major. A second advantage is that it provides a means of evaluating candidates to determine whether they need remedial work before continuing in the program.

Regardless of when and where assessment administration occurs, one or more people must be responsible for collecting and managing the assessment data. For PETE programs, NCATE requires two applications of each program assessment. ACSM exercise science accreditation considers assessment data from three key sources:

1. The accreditation exam.
2. Assessment of candidate clinical experience.
3. Evaluations from employers.

Because ACSM accreditation focuses on data from assessments occurring at the end of a program of study, sports medicine programs should consider building in additional decision points before candidates' clinical experience. Sport management programs also would benefit from adding decision points, because COSMA leaves decisions for candidate excellence to the discretion of each individual program's faculty. No matter the type, it's in the best interests of every program to track aggregated assessment data on a regular basis. Who should be responsible for collecting and managing that assessment data?

Resources and time become key determinants in selecting the best way to administer assessments, collect data and analyze results. Some programs might have adequate staff and/or graduate assistants available to input the assessment data into a data-management system. For programs that don't have that luxury, it's important to make the process as efficient and streamlined as possible.

In the section that follows, we offer an example of an effective, systematic model for managing assessment data. Within the model, each faculty member becomes a designated assessment coordinator for one particular program assessment. As such, his or her job is to administer and/or collect the data for the assigned assessment. Once data are collected, it is each individual assessment coordinator's responsibility to input that data into a program assessment database, to organize them into a summary table and to analyze them. All assessment coordinators meet at the end of each semester or academic year to share the analyses with program faculty members and, as a group, interpret the results. Once faculty members reach consensus on their interpretation of the data, they can determine what the program's next steps will be.

This model represents a systematic means of administering assessments, collecting data, conducting analysis and interpretation and developing an action plan ... as well as an efficient use of faculty time. Initial responsibility lies with each of the assessment coordinators; then, faculty members meet as a group to discuss data, interpret findings and make informed decisions.

Programs could enhance this assessment management model by tracking data over time, so that the information is more revealing and, therefore, trends can be interpreted appropriately. Data will always contain some outliers; examining program assessment data across several semesters will reflect a more accurate depiction of what's occurring. Programs that are submitting reports for external review (e.g., accreditation, national recognition) should consider requiring each of the assessment coordinators to prepare a draft summary as it applies to his or her designated assessment. Then, he or she can share the summary drafts with program faculty members and, after the discussion about the findings, can submit to the report compiler a revised draft that indicates consensus.

Developing an effective assessment management model is crucial to the program evaluation process. Program faculty members can choose to follow or modify the model presented above or create one that suits their program context, but they must implement some sort of data-tracking system.

Developing a filing system that backs up data in several formats also is a must. Storing all program assessment data — including actual assessment data and scoring results data — in both hard-copy and electronic formats, is the best way to ensure that important information is not lost. Multiple copies housed in different locations can provide the best way to prevent losing data.

Program Review Versus Program Report-Writing

Program faculty members must conduct a systematic program review (evaluation) before they can take on the task of writing a program report, be it for accreditation, national recognition, institutional effectiveness or annual department review. Program review/evaluation is the process by which program faculty members initiate change based on performance-based data; it's about the analysis and interpretation of data and decisions rendered based on those same data. In contrast, a program or self-study report is written communication that occurs in a designated format, addressing key questions about the program specific to whom and for what purpose the report is being written. Program evaluation must occur before a program report can be written. So, although they are different in nature, they are connected to each other.

As the program evaluation process occurs — especially during faculty dialogue while analyzing and interpreting data — it's critical for the program coordinator to designate someone as the recorder for each session. Someone must take accurate notes, which the group must affirm later so that a clear record of the interpretations and decisions made exists. The recorder role can be delegated to an administrative assistant, if available. Having someone outside the group serve as recorder will allow program faculty members to focus on the dialogue at hand. It also might be beneficial to audio-record the session for accuracy and review purposes. Written minutes from the sessions will provide the report compiler with an excellent source of documentation as he or she prepares to write various sections of the program report.

From an organizational perspective, it can be valuable to categorize evaluation meeting/session minutes according to content or sections specific to the program report template. The information files can be hard copy or electronic, depending on preference. All such documentation should be dated.

Finally, it's important to discuss how to get as much mileage as possible from assessment data. Faculty members often collect data simply to complete a SPA program report for national recognition. Because such valuable data are available, though, why not use them in other ways, as well? Program faculty members might use the data to make the case for adding a particular course to the curriculum. Or, assessment data might be used as part of the program's or department's institutional effectiveness (IE) plan. Perhaps the data provide strong support for a program change that faculty members want to initiate. Program faculty should be smart. It took a great deal of time, effort and hard work to gather and manage the data, conduct the analysis and interpret the data in an effort to bring about change. Program faculty should use the assessment data in as many ways as possible to contribute to improving the program.

Candidate Artifacts

Candidate artifacts are equally important for state-designated program reviews or institutional reviews for all academic programs. Artifacts provide genuine, authentic documentation of candidate competency specific to the program. Program faculty members should categorize candidate artifacts and keep them in an appropriate container or electronic storage system for easy access. Faculty members can use candidate artifacts to supplement yearly review portfolios, as well as for the purposes mentioned previously.

In addition to keeping examples of target-level performance by candidates, program faculty members should retain candidate work that represents both acceptable and unacceptable levels of performance, along with the scored rubric or scoring guide. That can help the program review team determine the program's rigor relative to the assessment. Faculty members must seek permission or approval to use candidate work in this manner, and identifying marks or names must be removed. Program faculty members should consider developing an approval form template that they can use across a variety of program assessments (see Appendix E). Each candidate would submit the form, documenting his or her consent, as part of the assessment task or assignment itself. Faculty members then can select the appropriate assessments for their purposes.

Although teacher candidate artifacts are not a part of the NASPE SPA program report, it's important for program faculty members to have these kinds of examples available. Candidate artifacts can be extremely important during the NCATE Board of Examiners' on-site visit during the accreditation process. The Board of Examiners team will consider these artifacts relative to candidate performance on selected program assessments. They can help the on-site team determine the quality of candidate work and gain valuable insights that might not otherwise be possible.

Setting a Timeline

The program coordinator is responsible for developing a comprehensive timeline for the program evaluation and/or program report submission process. The timeline should include designated tasks and initiatives, assigned responsibilities and projected deadlines as they relate to the program evaluation and/or report-writing processes. The program coordinator should determine the order in which the tasks ought to occur, because some tasks must be completed before others.

Once tasks are organized chronologically, the program coordinator should set deadlines, beginning with the final submission deadline and working backward. The last task in this process is to submit the final copy of the program report for accreditation, annual review or self-study. We recommend drafting a final version of the report no later than two weeks before the actual submission deadline to allow enough time in case technical or other difficulties arise. The keys are to plan ahead, allow extra time and be prepared for last-minute problems.

Developing a program evaluation timeline and adhering to the deadlines will keep program faculty members on track with what they need to do and when they need to do it to complete this complex endeavor in a timely fashion.

An Example of Curriculum Review & Redesign

We provide an illustration below of how the program evaluation process might be implemented within an academic program or department. The undergraduate program at the institution in this example offers a single degree: a Bachelor of Science in Kinesiology, but it does offer numerous program tracks leading to the degree under two general areas of specialization: teacher certification and exercise science. All program tracks share a kinesiology core. Except for general education requirements, however, each program track is specialized, dependent on the area of concentration. Program faculty members were required to submit a five-year program self-study report to the institution's undergraduate council. The process of curriculum review and redesign began two years earlier. What follows is the process undertaken to conduct a systematic review and redesign of the undergraduate programs to date. Most of the steps taken align with the program evaluation steps outlined in Chapter 1, although some modifications will be evident. Some deviations from the eight-step program evaluation process should be expected, because program faculty members undertake the evaluation process for many different reasons. Although the example does not explore management and organization aspects in detail, the process will be clear.

The undergraduate faculty members began with the questions (Step 1). No undergraduate philosophy statement had been created, so program faculty members discussed what was important to convey to degree candidates during the program of study, including faculty members' beliefs about kinesiology as it relates to curriculum. Initially, faculty members were divided into groups to share perceived beliefs with one another and to consolidate the beliefs into a list. Next, the faculty met as a whole and each group shared the beliefs it had discussed. The result was a set of core beliefs that all faculty members could buy into. The following undergraduate philosophy statement emerged as a result of those discussions:

> ... to promote professionalism within our students, faculty and staff
> that reflects the development of individuals who are educated based
> on principles and standards that promote the application of exercise,
> movement, teaching, research and service across the lifespan.

Next, program faculty members reviewed the IE outcomes and determined that they were still appropriate, in light of the new philosophy statement. Faculty members considered what graduates with a bachelor's degree in kinesiology from the department should know and be able to do by the time they completed their program of study.

What follows are the IE outcomes categories that guide all program tracks leading to the undergraduate kinesiology degree at the institution.

IE Outcome 1. In-Depth Knowledge and Skills
A. Demonstrate in-depth knowledge.
B. Demonstrate skills.

IE Outcome 2. Critical Thinking, Technology and Communication
A. Demonstrate ability to think and write critically.
B. Demonstrate ability to use technology.
C. Demonstrate ability to communicate effectively.

IE Outcome 3. Building a Fitness and Wellness Program
A. Demonstrate ability to build fitness and wellness programs for all populations.
B. Demonstrate ability to build a personal fitness and wellness program.

IE Outcome 4. Collaborative Skills and Professional Behaviors
A. Demonstrate ability to use collaborative skills.
B. Demonstrate professional behavior.

Because the institution offers only one undergraduate degree in kinesiology, program faculty members had to keep the outcomes broad enough to encompass all program tracks. Details specific to student learning outcomes are written for each of the two specialization areas.

Once it was determined that the department philosophy and alignment with IE outcomes were appropriate, the department chair formed three committees to provide input for the curriculum/program review and redesign:

1. Undergraduate Curriculum/Program Review Committee.
2. Undergraduate Physical Activity/Fitness Component Committee, comprised of two subcommittees:
   A. Kinesiology Health-Related Fitness Activity Core.
   B. Teacher Certification Physical Activity and Skill-Development Component.
3. Alumni, Graduating Seniors and Community Input Committee.

Chairs were appointed for each committee. The department chair's primary charge to all committees was to redesign program-track curricula in an effort to pursue national recognition or accreditation in the near future, and to encourage a standards-based curriculum. The goal was to pursue the following accreditations and/or certifications:

- Exercise science tracks:
  - ACSM Health Fitness Specialist Certification.
- Teacher-certification tracks:
  - All-level physical education teacher certification: NASPE Initial PETE National Recognition.
  - Adapted Physical Education National Standards (APENS) certification.

Based on its charge to attain national recognition, accreditation and/or certification in the targeted program tracks, the curriculum review committee employed the following process:

1. Committee members determined the national standards/elements on which to base the curricula. They included the ACSM Health Fitness Specialist Certification Standards, NASPE's Initial PETE Standards and the Adapted Physical Education National Standards.

2. Committee members developed a curriculum map for each program track (Standards & Elements/Course Matrix, see Appendix F). Those matrices provided the opportunity to review curricula to determine which national standards/elements were being addressed as primary, secondary and cursory foci within the program track courses currently in existence.

3. Committee members determined that all national standards/elements could align and be embedded within the current IE outcomes by developing matrices for each program track to illustrate the same (IE Outcomes/National Standards & Elements Matrix).

4. Concurrently, members of the physical activity/fitness component committee considered the teacher certification physical activity component and possible kinesiology and health-related core courses. Some potential courses were developed and piloted to obtain faculty and candidate feedback as to whether the courses would fit the new curricula.

5. Curriculum review committee members examined the standards & elements/course matrix carefully to determine how well current courses addressed the new standards and associated elements by program track, since former curricula were not standards-based and national standards for which accreditation would be sought had changed. That was done in the following manner:

   A. Program strengths were determined.

   B. Program weaknesses were uncovered.

C. Standards/elements where too much duplication was occurring were identified.

D. Standards/elements that were not being addressed or that were addressed insufficiently were identified.

6. Based on that review and input from the physical activity/fitness component committee, each program-track representative of the curriculum review committee — in consultation with faculty members most familiar with the program track — developed a draft redesigned curriculum track for his or her respective area.

7. Each program-track representative presented the proposed curriculum changes to the entire curriculum review committee to identify similarities and/or differences that might affect one another across program tracks based on proposed changes, including the kinesiology core.

8. Based on those discussions, each program-track representative finalized a first draft of the proposed curriculum changes and provided a strong justification for them.

9. The curriculum review committee presented the proposed curriculum redesign draft for each program track at a department meeting that featured open discussion. Concerns and positive input were recorded.

Meanwhile, the alumni, graduating seniors and community input committee members gathered data from alumni and graduating seniors that also would provide direction for the curriculum redesign. These data, in addition to data available based on IE outcomes, were examined to determine whether additional deficiencies existed that had to be addressed before developing final drafts of the curricula (Steps 2 & 3). Also, based on input gathered during the department meetings, committee members plan to seek advice and recommendations from community members/professionals with vested interests in the program graduates to review the proposals and provide further input into the process.

The curriculum review committee then plans to use all of that feedback from various constituencies to create final draft curricula to be presented to department faculty before submitting it to the university's curriculum committee.

Next, the undergraduate curriculum review committee will create a Standards & Elements/Course Assessment Matrix (see Appendix G). That will help in developing a set of program assessments and rubrics specific to each program track that align with and provide documentation of how each program is meeting the designated standards. (Some program assessments will be used across all program tracks.)

Once the new curricula take effect, program assessments will be administered and data will be tracked so that program faculty members will be able to discern how well candidates are performing (Step 3). Assessment coordinators will be designated for each program assessment, and program faculty members will collect, analyze and interpret data on a semi-annual or annual basis (Step 4). Based on that analysis and interpretation, program faculty members will render judgments about the new program tracks' quality (Step 5). Subsequently, after thorough discussion and dialogue, program faculty members will make explicit and informed decisions regarding programmatic and curriculum changes to improve program and candidate quality (Step 6). Faculty members then will implement the changes (Step 7). Most important, the department will continue the program evaluation process on a regular basis as program faculty members prepare to submit program reports for national recognition or accreditation, certification, unit reviews and institutional effectiveness (Step 8).

The preceding example illustrates just one way of implementing a systematic and continuous program evaluation — and program improvement — process. The process consumes a good amount of time, if done well, so it's important to build in enough time to attain the program's goal. The example above targeted the redesign of curricula to align with national standards in select disciplines, with the future goal of attaining national recognition, accreditation and certification. We hope that this example will help faculty members in other programs undertaking the program review process.

Conclusion

The process of program evaluation for program improvement is a time-consuming endeavor. Using the eight-step program evaluation process and recommendations offered in this chapter will give program faculty members a good start toward employing program evaluation as a continuous process. The program evaluation process is challenging, but, if managed appropriately, it can provide an effective means for ensuring program and candidate quality over time. Conducting program evaluation as a continuous process is the best way to improve program quality and candidate competency. Best wishes as you journey into continuous evaluation for program improvement!

References

Jewett, A.E., Bain, L.L., & Ennis, C.D. (1995). *The curriculum process in physical education*. Madison, WI: Brown and Benchmark.

Lund, J., & Tannehill, D. (2010). *Standards-based physical education curriculum development* (2nd ed.). Sudbury, MA: Jones and Bartlett.

Mager, R. (1984). *Preparing instructional objectives* (2nd ed.). Belmont, CA: David S. Lake Publishers.

Martin, R.J., & Judd, M. (2006). The NASPE/NCATE program report: From the reviewer's lens. *Journal of Physical Education, Recreation & Dance, 77*(3), 25-31.

Mizikaci, F. (2006). A systems approach to program evaluation model for quality in higher education. *Quality Assurance in Education, 14*(1), 37-53.

Morrow Jr., J.R., Jackson, A.W., Disch, J.G., & Mood, D.P. (2010). *Measurement and evaluation in human performance* (4th ed.). Champaign, IL: Human Kinetics.

National Association for Sport and Physical Education. (2004). *Moving into the future: National standards for physical education* (2nd ed.). Reston, VA: Author.

National Association for Sport and Physical Education. (2005, April). *Guidelines for initial physical education program reports*. Workshop materials presented at the annual AAHPERD Convention, Chicago, IL.

National Association for Sport and Physical Education. (2009). *National standards & guidelines for physical education teacher education* (3rd ed.). Reston, VA: Author.

National Association for Sport and Physical Education. (2010). *Pro-Link: Developing assessments and rubrics for NASPE/NCATE program reports*. Reston, VA: Author.

National Council for Accreditation of Teacher Education. (2008). *Professional standards for the accreditation of teacher preparation institutions*. Washington, DC: Author.

National Council for Accreditation of Teacher Education (2011a). *Program report for the initial preparation of physical education teachers (Option A)*. Retrieved September 6, 2011, from www.ncate.org/Standards/ProgramStandardsandReportForms/tabid/676/Default.aspx

National Council for Accreditation of Teacher Education (2011b). *Guidelines and procedures for the NCATE program review.* Retrieved September 6, 2011, from www.ncate.org/Accreditation/ProgramReview/GuidelinesAndProcedures/tabid/441/Default.aspx

National Council for Accreditation of Teacher Education (2011c). *New options for program review.* Retrieved September 27, 2011, from www.ncate.org/Accreditation/ProgramReview/GuidelinesAndProcedures/NewOptionsforProgramReview/tabid/650/Default.aspx

Oden, R.A. (2009). A college president's defense of accreditation. *New Directions for Higher Education, 145,* 37-45.

Rink, J.E. (2010). *Teaching physical education for learning* (6th ed.). Boston: McGraw-Hill.

Schön, D.A. (1983). *The reflective practitioner: How professionals think in action.* New York: Basic Books.

Senne, T.A. (2006). Writing the NASPE/NCATE program report: Process and practical suggestions. *Journal of Physical Education, Recreation, & Dance, 77*(3), 18-24, 31.

Wiggins, G. (1998). *Educative assessment: Designing assessments to inform and improve student performance.* San Francisco, CA: Jossey-Bass.

Appendix A

Documenting Course Grades as an Assessment of Candidate Content Knowledge

All SPAs will now accept grades in SPA-specific content courses as one content assessment. If programs choose to use course grades as one assessment, they must follow these guidelines. Grades can be used for Assessment #1 (if there is no state licensure test), Assessment #2 or one of the optional assessments.

Acceptable documentation required for programs using course grades:

1. Courses must be required for all candidates in the program; elective courses may not be used as evidence.
2. Faculty members may choose which courses will be used in this assessment. For example, they could select all courses in an academic major, they could select a cluster of courses that address a specific domain or they could select only one course, etc.
3. The documentation of course grades-based evidence must include curriculum requirements, including the course numbers of required courses. (a) For baccalaureate programs, documentation must be consistent with course listings provided in the Program of Study submitted in Section I of the program report. (b) If course grades are used as an assessment for a graduate level program that relies on coursework that may have been taken at another institution, the assessment must include the advising sheet that is used by the program to determine the sufficiency of courses taken by a candidate at another institution. The advising sheet must include specific information on required coursework and remediation required for deficiencies in the content acquirement of admitted candidates.
4. The grade evidence must be accompanied by the institution's grade policy or definitions of grades.

5. Grade data must be disaggregated by program level (e.g., baccalaureate and post-baccalaureate), grade level (e.g., middle grade and secondary), licensure category (e.g., history or social studies) and program site.

6. Syllabi **cannot** be submitted.

Format for Submission of Grades as a Course-Based Content Assessment

The following format is required for submission of grades as a course grade-based assessment under Section IV of the program report. For this specific assessment, these instructions take the place of the general instructions for submitting assessments cited at the beginning of Section IV.

Part 1. *Description of the assessment.* Provide a brief description of the courses and a rationale for selecting this particular set of courses. Provide a rationale for how these courses align with specific SPA standards, as well as an analysis of grade data included in the submission. (Limit to two pages.)

NOTE: **If course grades are used as an assessment for a graduate-level program that relies on coursework that may have been taken at another institution, the report must include the advising sheet that the program uses to determine the sufficiency of courses taken by a candidate at another institution.**

Part 2. *Alignment with SPA standards.* This part must include a matrix that shows alignment of courses with specific SPA standards. Faculty members may choose one of the following two examples; one is organized by course, the other is organized by SPA standard. Brief course descriptions should be included if the course title does not identify the course content.

A graduate-level program that relies on coursework that may have been taken at another institution must show alignment between the SPA standards and the program's advising sheet that is used to determine the sufficiency of courses taken by a candidate at another institution.

Example 1: Alignment Matrix Organized by Course

Course Name & Number	SPA Standard(s) Addressed by Course	Brief Description of How the Course Meets Cited Standards (if Course Title Is Unclear)
MATH 150: Discrete Mathematics	9.5, 9.7, 13.1, 13.2, 13.3	

Example 2: Alignment Matrix Organized by SPA Standard

SPA Standard(s) Addressed by Course	Course Name & Number	Brief Description of How the Course Meets Cited Standards (if Course Title Is Unclear)
NCTE 3.5	Young Adult Literature 203	
NCTE 3.6	English 105	

Part 3. *Grade Policy and Minimum Expectation.* The program must submit grading policies that are used by the institution or program and the minimum expectation for candidate grades (e.g., all candidates must achieve a C or better in all selected coursework).

Part 4. *Data table(s).* Data tables must provide, at minimum, the grade distributions and mean course grades for candidates in the selected courses. **NOTE: The "n" in the data table/s for each year or semester must be relatively consistent with the numbers of candidates and completers reported in Attachment A to Section I.** Large inconsistencies between the two data sets must be explained in a note included with the data table(s).

NOTE: If course grades are used as an assessment for a graduate-level program that relies on coursework that may have been taken at another institution, the program may provide data as candidates' grade point average across all courses listed on program advising sheet or transcript analysis form.

Part 4. Sample Data Tables

Example 1. Candidates' Grades in Required Mathematics Courses Secondary Math Education Candidates Baccalaureate Program

	2004-2005		2005-2006		2006-2007	
	Average course grade and (range)*	% of candidates meeting minimum expectation	Average course grade and (range)	% of candidates meeting minimum expectation	Average course grade and (range)	% of candidates meeting minimum expectation
Math 101	3.75 (3.0–3.9)	100	3.75 (3.0–3.9)	92	3.75 (3.0–3.9)	97
Math 203	3.3 (3.0 – 3.5)	95	3.3 (3.0 – 3.5)	100	3.3 (3.0 – 3.5)	88
Math 305	3.4 (3.2 – 3.7)	87	3.4 (3.2 – 3.7)	89	3.4 (3.2 – 3.7)	100

Example 2. Mean GPA in Science Major Courses for Candidates Admitted to MAT Program Secondary Science Education Candidates

SPA Standard(s) Addressed by Course	Course Name & Number	Brief Description of How the Course Meets Cited Standards (if Course Title Is Unclear)
NCTE 3.5	Young Adult Literature 203	
NCTE 3.6	English 105	

Reprinted with permission from National Council for Accreditation of Teacher Education, www.ncate.org.

Appendix B

Program Report for the Initial Preparation of Physical Education Teachers Option A

American Alliance for Health, Physical Education, Recreation and Dance

National Association for Sport and Physical Education (NASPE)
(2008 Standards)

NATIONAL COUNCIL FOR ACCREDITATION OF TEACHER EDUCATION

Cover Sheet

1. Institution Name

2. City/State

3. Date submitted

MM   DD   YYYY

☐ / ☐ / ☐

4. **Report Compiler's Information:**

Name:

Phone: Ext.

( ) -

E-mail:

5. **NCATE Coordinator's Information:**

Name:

Phone: Ext.

( ) -

E-mail:

6. Name of institution's program

7. NCATE Category

8. Grade levels[1] for which candidates are being prepared

9. **Program Type**
   - ▪ First teaching license

10. **Degree**
    - ▪ Baccalaureate
    - ▪ Post Baccalaureate
    - ▪ Master's, initial certification

(1) e.g. K-6, K-12, 7-12

11. Is this program offered at more than one site?

⚫ Yes

⚫ No

12. If your answer is "Yes" to above question, list the sites at which the program is offered

13. Title of the state license for which candidates are prepared

14. Program report status:

⚫ First Submission for review

⚫ Response to National Recognition With Conditions

⚫ Response to One of the Following Decisions: Further Development Required or Recognition With Probation

15. Is your unit seeking

⚫ NCATE accreditation for the first time (initial accreditation)

⚫ Continuing NCATE accreditation

16. State Licensure requirement for national recognition:

If using Praxis as your state licensure exam for PETE, the appropriate, preferred form is Praxis 0091, Physical Education Content Exam. If your state requires the combined Health and Physical Education Praxis exam, that will be acceptable.

NCATE requires 80% of the program completers who have taken the test to pass the applicable state licensure test for the content field, if the state has a testing requirement. Test information and data must be reported in Section IV. Does your state require such a test?

⚫ Yes

⚫ No

SECTION I - CONTEXT

1. Description of any state or institutional policies that may influence the application of AAHPERD/NASPE standards. (Response limited to 4,000 characters)

2. Description of the field and clinical experiences required for the program, including the number of hours for early field experiences and the number of hours/weeks for student teaching or internships. (Response limited to 8,000 characters)

3. Please attach files to describe a program of study that outlines the courses and experiences required for candidates to complete the program. The program of study must include course titles. (This information may be provided as an attachment from the college catalog or as a student advisement sheet.)

4. This system will not permit you to include tables or graphics in text fields. Therefore any tables or charts must be attached as files here. The title of the file should clearly indicate the content of the file. Word documents, pdf files, and other commonly used file formats are acceptable.

5. Candidate Information

Directions: Provide three years of data on candidates enrolled in the program and completing the program, beginning with the most recent academic year for which numbers have been tabulated. Report the data separately for the levels/tracks (e.g., baccalaureate, post-baccalaureate, master's initial licensure) being addressed in this report. Data must also be reported separately for programs offered at multiple sites. Update academic years (column 1) as appropriate for your data span. Create additional tables as necessary.

Program:		
Academic Year	**# of Candidates Enrolled in the Program**	**# of Program Completers[2]**

(2) NCATE uses the Title II definition for program completers. Program completers are persons who have met all the requirements of a state-approved teacher preparation program. Program completers include all those who are documented as having met such requirements. Documentation may take the form of a degree, institutional certificate, program credential, transcript, or other written proof of having met the program's requirements.

6. Faculty Information

Directions: Complete the following information for each faculty member responsible for professional coursework, clinical supervision, or administration in this program.

Faculty Member Name	
Highest Degree, Field, & University[3]	
Assignment: Indicate the role of the faculty member[4]	
Faculty Rank[5]	
Tenure Track	☞ YES
Scholarship[6]**, Leadership in Professional Associations, and Service** [7]**:List up to 3 major contributions in the past 3 years**[8]	
Teaching or other professional experience in P-12 schools[9]	

(3) e.g., PhD in Curriculum & Instruction, University of Nebraska.
(4) e.g., faculty, clinical supervisor, department chair, administrator
(5) e.g., professor, associate professor, assistant professor, adjunct professor, instructor
(6) Scholarship is defined by NCATE as systematic inquiry into the areas related to teaching, learning, and the education of teachers and other school personnel. Scholarship includes traditional research and publication as well as the rigorous and systematic study of pedagogy, and the application of current research findings in new settings. Scholarship further presupposes submission of one's work for professional review and evaluation.
(7) Service includes faculty contributions to college or university activities, schools, communities, and professional associations in ways that are consistent with the institution and unit's mission.
(8) e.g., officer of a state or national association, article published in a specific journal, and an evaluation of a local school program.
(9) Briefly describe the nature of recent experience in P-12 schools (e.g. clinical supervision, in-service training, teaching in a PDS) indicating the discipline and grade level of the assignment(s). List current P-12 licensure or certification(s) held, if any.

SECTION II - LIST OF ASSESSMENTS

1. In this section, list the 6-8 assessments that are being submitted as evidence for meeting the AAHPERD/NASPE standards elements. All programs must provide a minimum of six assessments. If your state does not require a state licensure test in the content area, you must substitute an assessment that documents candidate attainment of content knowledge in #1 below. For each assessment, indicate the type or form of the assessment and when it is administered in the program. (Response limited to 250 characters each field)

Type and Number of Assessment	Name of Assessment [10]	Type or Form of Assessment [11]	When the Assessment Is Administered [12]
Assessment #1: Licensure assessment, or other content-based assessment (required)			
Assessment #2: Content knowledge in physical education (required)			
Assessment #3: Candidate ability to plan instruction (required)			
Assessment #4: Internship or clinical experiences (required)			
Assessment #5: Candidate effect on student learning (required)			
Assessment #6: Additional assessment that addresses AAHPERD/NASPE standards (required)			

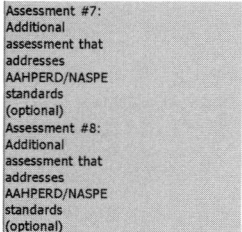

| Assessment #7: Additional assessment that addresses AAHPERD/NASPE standards (optional) | |
| Assessment #8: Additional assessment that addresses AAHPERD/NASPE standards (optional) | |

(10) Identify assessment by title used in the program; refer to Section IV for further information on appropriate assessment to include.

(11) Identify the type of assessment (e.g., essay, case study, project, comprehensive exam, reflection, state licensure test, portfolio).

(12) Indicate the point in the program when the assessment is administered (e.g., admission to the program, admission to student teaching/internship, required courses [specify course title and numbers], or completion of the program).

SECTION III - RELATIONSHIP OF ASSESSMENT TO STANDARDS

For each AAHPERD/NASPE standard on the chart below, identify the assessment(s) in Section II that address the standard. One assessment may apply to multiple AAHPERD/NASPE standards.

1. Standard 1: Scientific and Theoretical Knowledge

Physical education teacher candidates know and apply discipline-specific scientific and theoretical concepts critical to the development of physically educated individuals

	#1	#2	#3	#4	#5	#6	#7	#8
1.1 Describe and apply physiological and biomechanical concepts related to skillful movement, physical activity and fitness.	☐	☐	☐	☐	☐	☐	☐	☐
1.2 Describe and apply motor learning and psychological/behavioral theory related to skillful movement, physical activity and fitness.	☐	☐	☐	☐	☐	☐	☐	☐
1.3 Describe and apply motor development theory and principles related to skillful movement, physical activity and fitness.	☐	☐	☐	☐	☐	☐	☐	☐
1.4 Identify historical, philosophical and social perspectives of physical education issues and legislation.	☐	☐	☐	☐	☐	☐	☐	☐
1.5 Analyze and correct critical elements of motor skills and performance concepts.	☐	☐	☐	☐	☐	☐	☐	☐

2. Standard 2: Skill-Based and Fitness Based Competence*

Physical education teacher candidates are physically educated individuals with the knowledge and skills necessary to demonstrate competent movement performance and health-enhancing fitness as delineated in the NASPE K – 12 Standards.

	#1	#2	#3	#4	#5	#6	#7	#8
2.1 Demonstrate personal competence in motor skill performance for a variety of physical activities and movement patterns.	☐	☐	☐	☐	☐	☐	☐	☐
2.2 Achieve and maintain a health-enhancing level of fitness throughout the program.	☐	☐	☐	☐	☐	☐	☐	☐
2.3 Demonstrate performance concepts related to skillful movement in a variety of physical activities.	☐	☐	☐	☐	☐	☐	☐	☐

*Without discrimination against those with disabilities, physical education teacher candidates with special needs are allowed and encouraged to use a variety of accommodations and/or modifications to demonstrate competent movement and performance concepts (e.g., modified/adapted equipment, augmented communication devices, multi-media devices) and fitness (e.g., weight training programs, exercise logs).

3. Standard 3: Planning and Implementation

Physical education teacher candidates plan and implement developmentally appropriate learning experiences aligned with local, state and national standards to address the diverse needs of all students.

	#1	#2	#3	#4	#5	#6	#7	#8
3.1 Design and implement short-term and long-term plans that are linked to program and instructional goals as well as a variety of student needs.	☐	☐	☐	☐	☐	☐	☐	☐
3.2 Develop and implement appropriate (e.g., measurable, developmentally appropriate, performance-based) goals and objectives aligned with local, state and /or national standards.	☐	☐	☐	☐	☐	☐	☐	☐
3.3 Design and implement content that is aligned with lesson objectives.	☐	☐	☐	☐	☐	☐	☐	☐
3.4 Plan for and manage resources to provide active, fair and equitable learning experiences.	☐	☐	☐	☐	☐	☐	☐	☐
3.5 Plan and adapt instruction for diverse student needs, adding specific accommodations and/or modifications								

for student exceptionalities.

	#1	#2	#3	#4	#5	#6	#7	#8
3.6 Plan and implement progressive and sequential instruction that addresses the diverse needs of all students.								
3.7 Demonstrate knowledge of current technology by planning and implementing learning experiences that require students to appropriately use technology to meet lesson objectives.								

4. Standard 4: Instructional Delivery and Management
Physical education teacher candidates use effective communication and pedagogical skills and strategies to enhance student engagement and learning.

	#1	#2	#3	#4	#5	#6	#7	#8
4.1 Demonstrate effective verbal and non-verbal communication skills across a variety of instructional formats								
4.2 Implement effective demonstrations, explanations, and instructional cues and prompts to link physical activity concepts to appropriate learning experiences.								
4.3 Provide effective instructional feedback for skill acquisition, student learning and motivation.								
4.4 Recognize the changing dynamics of the environment and adjust instructional tasks based on student responses.								
4.5 Use managerial rules, routines and transitions to create and maintain a safe and effective learning environment.								
4.6 Implement strategies to help students demonstrate responsible personal and social behaviors in a productive learning environment.								

5. Standard 5: Impact on Student Learning
Physical education teacher candidates use assessments and reflection to foster student learning and inform decisions about instructions.

	#1	#2	#3	#4	#5	#6	#7	#8
5.1 Select or create appropriate assessments that will measure student achievement of goals and objectives.								
5.2 Use appropriate assessments to evaluate student learning before, during and after instruction.								
5.3 Use the reflective cycle to implement change in teacher performance, student learning and/or instruction goals and decisions.								

6. Standard 6: Professionalism
Physical education teacher candidates demonstrate dispositions that are essential to becoming effective professionals.

	#1	#2	#3	#4	#5	#6	#7	#8
6.1 Demonstrate behaviors that are consistent with the belief that all students can become physically educated individuals.								
6.2 Participate in activities that enhance collaboration and lead to professional growth and development.								
6.3 Demonstrate behaviors that are consistent with the professional ethics of highly qualified teachers.								
6.4 Communicate in ways that convey respect and sensitivity.								

SECTION IV - EVIDENCE FOR MEETING STANDARDS

DIRECTIONS: The 6-8 key assessments listed in Section II must be documented and discussed in Section IV. Taken as a whole, the assessments must demonstrate candidate mastery of the SPA standards and elements. The key assessments should be required of all candidates. Assessments and scoring guides and data charts should be aligned with the SPA standards. This means that the concepts in the SPA standards and elements should be apparent in the assessments and in the scoring guides to the same depth, breadth and specificity as in the SPA standards and elements. Data tables should also be aligned with the SPA standards and elements. The data should be presented, in general, at the same level it is collected. For example, if a rubric collects data on 10 elements [each relating to specific SPA standard(s)], then the data chart should report the data on each of the elements rather that reporting a cumulative score.

In the description of each assessment below, the SPA has identified potential assessments that would be appropriate. Assessments have been organized into the following three areas to be aligned with the elements in NCATE's unit standard 1:
• Content knowledge (Assessments 1 and 2)
• Pedagogical and professional knowledge, skills and dispositions (Assessments 3 and 4)
• Focus on student learning (Assessment 5)

Note that, in some disciplines, content knowledge may include or be inextricable from professional knowledge. If this is the case, assessments that combine content and professional knowledge may be considered "content knowledge" assessments for the purpose of this report.

For each assessment, the compiler should prepare one document that includes the following items:

(1) A two-page narrative that includes the following:
  a. A brief description of the assessment and its use in the program;
  b. A description of how this assessment specifically aligns with the standards and elements it is cited for in Section III. Cite SPA standards/elements by number (e.g.,1.1 or 1.2);
  c. A brief analysis of the data findings;
  d. An interpretation of how that data provides evidence for meeting standards/elements, indicating the specific SPA standards and elements by number (e.g.,1.1 or 1.2 etc);

and

(2) Assessment documentation
  e. The assessment tool itself or a rich description of the assessment (often the directions given to candidates);
  f. The scoring guide for the assessment; and
  g. Charts that provide candidate data derived from the assessment.

The responses for e, f and g above should be limited to the equivalent of five text pages each. However, in some cases, assessment instruments or scoring guides may go beyond five pages.

Note: As much as possible, combine all of the files for one assessment into a single file. That is, create one file for Assessment #4 that includes the two-page narrative (items a – d above), the assessment itself (item e above), the scoring guide (item f above, and the data chart (item g above). Each attachment should be no larger than 2 mb. Do not include candidate work or syllabi. There is a limit of 20 attachments for the entire report, so it is crucial that you combine files as much as possible.

1. State licensure tests or professional examinations of content knowledge. AAHPERD/NASPE standards addressed in this entry could include but are not limited to Standard 1. If your state does not require licensure tests or professional examinations in the content area, data from another assessment must be presented to document candidate attainment of content knowledge. (Assessment Required)

Provide assessment information (items 1. a, b, c, d and 2.e, f, g) as outlined in the directions for Section IV. A complete description of the assessment should be included (format of the exam, content area sub-scores).

2. Assessment of content knowledge in the field of physical education. AAHPERD/NASPE standards addressed in this assessment could include but are not limited to Standards 1 and 2. Examples of assessments include comprehensive examinations, portfolios; health- related fitness assessments, assessments of fundamental movement skills; and assessments of performance-competency and game play. (Assessment Required)

Provide assessment information (items 1. a, b, c, d and 2.e, f, g) as outlined in the directions for Section IV.

3. Assessment that demonstrates candidates can effectively plan classroom-based instruction. AAHPERD/NASPE standards that could be addressed in this assessment include but are not limited to Standard 3. Examples of assessments include the evaluation of candidates' abilities to develop lesson or unit plans, individualized education plans, needs assessments or intervention plans. (Assessment Required)

Provide assessment information (items 1. a, b, c, d and 2.e, f, g) as outlined in the directions for Section IV.

4. Assessment that demonstrates candidates' knowledge, skills and dispositions are applied effectively in practice. AAHPERD/NASPE standards that could be addressed in this assessment include Standards 3 and 4. The assessment instrument used in the internship or other clinical experiences should be submitted. (Assessment Required)

Provide assessment information (items 1. a, b, c, d and 2.e, f, g) as outlined in the directions for Section IV.

5. Assessment that demonstrates candidate effects on student learning and the creation of supportive learning environments for student learning. AAHPERD/NASPE standards that could be addressed in this assessment include but are not limited to Standard 5. Examples of assessments include those based on student work samples, (IEPs), case studies or implemented unit plans. (Assessment Required)

Provide assessment information (items 1. a, b, c, d and 2.e, f, g) as outlined in the directions for Section IV.

6. Additional assessment that addresses AAHPERD/NASPE standards. Examples of assessments include evaluations of field experiences, case studies, teacher candidate work sample, IEPs or other key assessment. (Assessment Required)

Provide assessment information (items 1. a, b, c, d and 2.e, f, g) as outlined in the directions for Section IV.

7. **Additional assessment that addresses AAHPERD/NASPE standards.** Examples of assessments include evaluations of field experiences, teacher candidate work sample, case studies, IEPs, or other appropriate assessments. (optional)

Provide assessment information (items 1. a,b,c,d and 2.e,f,g) as outlined in the directions for Section IV

8. **Additional assessment that addresses AAHPERD/NASPE standards.** Examples of assessments include evaluations of field experiences, case studies, portfolio tasks and licensure tests not reported in #1. (optional)

Provide assessment information (items 1. a,b,c,d and 2.e,f,g) as outlined in the directions for Section IV

SECTION V - USE OF ASSESSMENT RESULTS TO IMPROVE PROGRAM

1. **Evidence must be presented in this section that assessment results have been analyzed and have been or will be used to improve candidate performance and strengthen the program. This description should not link improvements to individual assessments but, rather, it should summarize principal findings (data) from the evidence, the faculty's interpretation of those findings, and changes made in (or planned for) the program as a result. Describe the steps program faculty has taken to use information from assessments for improvement of both candidate performance and the program. This information should be organized around (1) content knowledge, (2) professional and pedagogical knowledge, skill, and dispositions, and (3) student learning.**

(Response limited to 12,000 characters)

SECTION VI - FOR REVISED REPORTS OR RESPONSE TO CONDITIONS REPORTS ONLY

1. **For Revised Reports: Describe what changes or additions have been made to address the standards that were not met in the original submission. Provide new responses to questions and/or new documents to verify the changes described in this section. Specific instructions for preparing a Revised Report are available on the NCATE web site at http://www.ncate.org/Accreditation/ProgramReview/ProgramReportSubmission/RevisedProgramReports/tabid/453/Default.aspx**

For Response to Conditions Reports: Describe what changes or additions have been made to address the conditions cited in the original recognition report. Provide new responses to questions and/or new documents to verify the changes described in this section. Specific instructions for preparing a Response to Conditions Report are available on the NCATE web site at http://www.ncate.org/Accreditation/ProgramReview/ProgramReportSubmission/ResponsetoConditionsReport/tabid/454/Default.aspx

(Response limited to 24,000 characters.)

Please click "Next"

This is the end of the report. Please click "Next" to proceed.

Reprinted with permission from National Council for Accreditation of Teacher Education, www.ncate.org.

Appendix C

NASPE Initial PETE Elements/Assessment Table

NASPE Initial PETE Elements/Assessment Table

Standard 1: Scientific and Theoretical Knowledge
Physical education teacher candidates know and apply discipline-specific scientific and theoretical concepts critical to the development of physically educated individuals.

Elements – Teacher candidates will:	Assessments
1.1 Describe and apply physiological and biomechanical concepts related to skillful movement, physical activity and fitness.	
1.2 Describe and apply motor learning and psychological/behavioral theory related to skillful movement, physical activity and fitness.	
1.3 Describe and apply motor development theory and principles related to skillful movement, physical activity and fitness.	
1.4 Identify historical, philosophical and social perspectives of physical education issues and legislation.	
1.5 Analyze and correct critical elements of motor skills and performance concepts.	

The two most comprehensive assessments for Standard 1 are:

1._____

2._____

Standard 2: Skill-Based and Fitness-Based Competence*
Physical education teacher candidates are physically educated individuals with the knowledge and skills necessary to demonstrate competent movement performance and health-enhancing fitness as delineated in the NASPE K–12 Standards.

Elements – Teacher candidates will:	Assessments
2.1 Demonstrate personal competence in motor skill performance for a variety of physical activities and movement patterns.	
2.2 Achieve and maintain a health-enhancing level of fitness throughout the program.	
2.3 Demonstrate performance concepts related to skillful movement in a variety of physical activities.	

* Without discrimination against those with disabilities, physical education teacher candidates with special needs are allowed and encouraged to use a variety of accommodations and/or modifications (e.g., modified/adapted equipment, augmented communication devices, multimedia devices) to demonstrate competent movement and performance concepts and fitness.

The two most comprehensive assessments for Standard 2 are:

1._____

2._____

Standard 3: Planning and Implementation
Physical education teacher candidates plan and implement developmentally appropriate learning experiences aligned with local, state and national standards to address the diverse needs of all students.

Elements – Teacher candidates will:	Assessments
3.1 Design and implement short- and long-term plans that are linked to program and instructional goals, as well as a variety of student needs.	
3.2 Develop and implement appropriate (e.g., measurable, developmentally appropriate, performance-based) goals and objectives aligned with local, state and /or national standards.	
3.3 Design and implement content that is aligned with lesson objectives.	
3.4 Plan for and manage resources to provide active, fair and equitable learning experiences.	
3.5 Plan and adapt instruction for diverse student needs, adding specific accommodations and/or modifications for student exceptionalities.	
3.6 Plan and implement progressive and sequential instruction that addresses the diverse needs of all students.	
3.7 Demonstrate knowledge of current technology by planning and implementing learning experiences that require students to use technology appropriately to meet lesson objectives.	

The two most comprehensive assessments for Standard 3 are:

1._____

2._____

Standard 4: Instructional Delivery and Management
Physical education teacher candidates use effective communication and pedagogical skills and strategies to enhance student engagement and learning.

Elements – Teacher candidates will:	Assessments
4.1 Demonstrate effective verbal and non-verbal communication skills across a variety of instructional formats.	
4.2 Implement effective demonstrations, explanations and instructional cues and prompts to link physical activity concepts to appropriate learning experiences.	
4.3 Provide effective instructional feedback for skill acquisition, student learning and motivation.	
4.4 Recognize the changing dynamics of the environment and adjust instructional tasks based on student responses.	
4.5 Use managerial rules, routines and transitions to create and maintain a safe and effective learning environment.	
4.6 Implement strategies to help students demonstrate responsible personal and social behaviors in a productive learning environment.	

The two most comprehensive assessments for Standard 4 are:

1._____

2._____

Standard 5: Impact on Student Learning
Physical education teacher candidates use assessments and reflection to foster student learning and inform instructional decisions.

Elements – Teacher candidates will:	Assessments
5.1 Select or create appropriate assessments that will measure student achievement of goals and objectives.	
5.2 Use appropriate assessments to evaluate student learning before, during and after instruction.	
5.3 Use the reflective cycle to implement change in teacher performance, student learning and/or instructional goals and decisions.	

The two most comprehensive assessments for Standard 5 are:

1._____

2._____

Standard 6: Professionalism
Physical education teacher candidates demonstrate dispositions that are essential to becoming effective professionals.

Elements – Teacher candidates will:	Assessments
6.1 Demonstrate behaviors that are consistent with the belief that all students can become physically educated individuals.	
6.2 Participate in activities that enhance collaboration and lead to professional growth and development.	
6.3 Demonstrate behaviors that are consistent with the professional ethics of highly qualified teachers.	
6.4 Communicate in ways that convey respect and sensitivity.	

The two most comprehensive assessments for Standard 6 are:

1._____

2._____

Appendix D

NCATE Assessment 3 – Lesson Plan

Partial Example

(Modified and used with permission from Stevie Chepko, Ed.D., Winthrop University)

NCATE Assessment 3 – Lesson Plan

Authors' note: *This assessment package (Attachments a, b and c) has been modified. It is used with the permission of Stevie Chepko, Ed.D., Winthrop University. Our thanks to her for her willingness to share for the benefit of other PETE programs.*

This example is provided to show programs how to include documentation of NASPE Initial PETE Standards and Elements within the following three documents as part of Section IV of the NASPE/NCATE Program Report Template:

- Assessment (or assignment).
- Scoring guide or rubric.
- Data summary table.

Identification of NASPE Initial PETE Standards and Elements in each of the above documents should be found in every assessment bundle that appears in Section IV of the NASPE/NCATE Program Report.

To view the example NCATE Assessment 3 Lesson Plan document in its original form (as posted in the SPA Library), visit www.ncate.org/Accreditation/ProgramReview/ProgramReviewResources/SPAAssessmentLibrary/tabid/460/Default.aspx.

ATTACHMENT 3a – Lesson Plan

Description of Assignment

Contextual Information

On the lesson plan form, you must include the required contextual information about the class. This information includes size of the class, grade level, number of students in the class, equipment needed for the class and the overall theme of the lesson.

Lesson Objectives

All effective lessons begin with the creation of objectives that will lead to the meeting of unit-level goals and state/national standards. Lesson objectives are central to planning and implementing effective lessons. All objectives that you create should meet the following criteria:

1. Objectives are performance-based and measurable. (NASPE 3.2)
2. Objectives are developmentally appropriate for the grade/age levels. (NASPE 3.2)
3. Objectives are congruent with unit, state and national standards. (NASPE 3.2)
4. All lessons should include objective(s) in the affective, motor and cognitive domains.
5. All objectives include three of the four components (action verb, content, criteria or conditions).
6. Each lesson has multiple objectives.
7. Objectives address a variety of student needs/interests.
8. At least one objective in each lesson should link directly to increasing opportunities for students to demonstrate responsible personal and social behaviors. (NASPE 4.6)

Teacher Objectives

For each lesson, you must identify behaviors that you would like to improve in your teaching. These teacher objectives are about how you will improve your effectiveness by making specific changes in your presentation or interactions with students. That includes behaviors concerning feedback to students, your movement in the classroom, various managerial skills, and improving communication skills or other behaviors that you believe will enhance your teaching effectiveness. This is the first step in becoming a reflective practitioner.

1. Teacher objectives are stated in terms of expected teacher behaviors.
2. Teacher objectives are specific and measurable.

Instructional Plan

The instructional plan is central to the planning process. In this part of the lesson plan, you outline the scope and sequence of the lesson. Part of the evaluation of your teaching effectiveness will be your ability to implement the instruction plan. Listed below are key components of the instructional plan.

1. Lesson has an identifiable opening (instant activity/preview/etc.).
2. Learning/practice tasks are linked directly to learning objectives. (NASPE 3.3)
3. Learning/practice tasks are explained in detail, with organizational diagrams of the classroom environment.
4. Learning/practice tasks are progressive and sequential. (NASPE 3.6)
5. All learning/practice tasks provide active, fair and equitable learning environments. (NASPE 3.4)
6. Learning/practice tasks are psychologically and physically safe and appropriate for all students. (NASPE 3.5)
7. Demonstrations of skills or concepts are planned for and implemented during the lesson. (NASPE 4.2)
8. For each skill/concept taught, appropriate instructional cues and prompts are identified and used. (NASPE 4.2)
9. Plans are identified for adapting and accommodating high- and low-performing students or students with special needs, and the plan is implemented. (NASPE 3.5)
10. If appropriate for lesson objectives, student use of technology is planned and implemented to accomplish lesson/unit goals. At least one lesson per unit includes technology. (NASPE 3.7)
11. Practice tasks include refinements, extensions, modifications (if applicable) and applications.
12. Practice tasks allow for individual differences and adaptations in starting/ending points, equipment or grouping. (NASPE 3.5)

Transition/Management

To increase the available instruction time, you must plan for efficient transitions in a lesson and manage students and resources effectively.

1. Transitions are planned for, described clearly and implemented effectively to increase instruction/activity time. (NASPE 4.5)
2. Beginning and ending signals are identified and used.
3. Routines are established for tasks such as equipment distribution/collection, grouping/partnering, water breaks, etc. (NASPE 4.5)
4. Rules are established and enforced to ensure an effective and equitable learning environment. (NASPE 4.5)
5. The number of transitions is minimized.

Assessment

To determine whether you have met your objectives, you must plan for and implement both formal and informal assessments. Assessments can include formal pre/post assessments or simple checks for understanding throughout the lesson. All lessons should include some type of assessments so that you can determine whether your objectives were met or you need to readdress the objectives in later lessons.

1. Assessments are aligned with and appropriate for lesson objectives and developmental levels. (NASPE 5.1)
2. If formal assessment is conducted, a plan for recording the data is established and the protocol is followed.
3. Assessments are appropriate measures of student achievement of goals/objectives. (NASPE 5.1)
4. Assessments (informal or formal) occur throughout the lesson and adjustments to lesson are made based on assessments. (NASPE 5.2)

Closure

Every lesson must have closure. Your lesson plan must include a complete description of how you will close the lesson. Remember to remind students of key skill cues or concepts taught during the lesson and preview the next lesson.

1. Plan and implement a closure that summarizes the lesson's key points, checks for student understanding and previews the next lesson.
2. Plan and implement a closure that is aligned directly with lesson objectives.

Safety/Technology Use/Special Considerations

Physical education teachers have students moving through large spaces often with equipment. It's the responsibility of every teacher to ensure the safety of students in the classroom, but it's particularly important for physical educators. In this section, you will identify how you have ensured the safety of students in your class. In addition to identifying any safety concerns, you should document any use of technology by students in this section.

1. Safety issues are planned for and strategies are used to ensure students' safety. Examples include ensuring that the space is clear of obstacles, that the space is large enough for students to move freely and that rules are established for the appropriate use of equipment. (NASPE 4.5)
2. Students' use of technology — including pedometers, video cameras, watches and other forms of appropriate technology — is identified in the plan. (NASPE 3.7)

Resources

All effective teachers develop learning experiences based on the best practices and research in the discipline. Those resources can include textbooks, appropriate Web sites and lesson plans created and shared by other professionals in the field. In this section, you should cite — using APA format — which resources you use for developing your lesson.

1. Resources are identified, including page numbers and/or Web addresses.
2. Resources are identified using APA citation rules.

ATTACHMENT 3b
Lesson Plan Rubric

Name of Student: _____   Date: _____

Course: _____

Section of Lesson Plan	Unacceptable (1 point)	Acceptable (2 points)	Target (3 points)	Total Score
Contextual Information	At least two components of the required contextual information (e.g., class size, equipment needed, grade level, theme of lesson) are missing.	All required components of the contextual information are included.	All required components of the contextual information are included, and both a movement concept and skills themes are identified.	
Lesson Objectives				
Objectives are performance-based and measurable, and they contain three of the four components (action verb, content, criteria and conditions). (NASPE 3.2)	Lesson objectives use terms such as "understand" or "learn," which are neither performance-based nor measureable. Only action verbs and content are identified in all of the objectives.	Lesson objectives use measurable action verbs such as "demonstrate," "apply" or "identify," and are performance-based. A minority of the objectives identify either a condition or criteria.	Lesson objectives are performance-based and measurable, and are written with clarity and specificity. All objectives contain either a condition or criteria.	
Objectives are developmentally appropriate for the grade/age levels. (NASPE 3.2)	Lesson objectives are incongruent with students' grade or developmental level by being too easy or too difficult. Content identified in objectives is inappropriate for students' developmental level.	Lesson objectives are congruent with students' grade and developmental levels. Content identified in objectives is appropriate for students' developmental level.	Lesson objectives are congruent with students' grade and developmental levels. Objectives identify key content that is aligned with students' developmental level.	

Lesson Objectives	Unacceptable (1 point)	Acceptable (2 points)	Target (3 points)	Score
Lesson has multiple objectives, with at least one objective in each domain of learning.	Lesson plan includes objectives in just one or two domains. Fewer than three objectives are identified for the lesson.	Lesson includes multiple objectives for the lesson and at least one objective in each of the domains.	Lesson includes more than one objective in at least two of the three domains and at least one objective in each domain.	
At least one objective in the affective domain is linked to students' developing responsible social and personal behaviors. (NASPE 4.6)	No objectives are written in the affective domain or are not linked to responsible social and personal behavior.	At least one objective is written in the affective domain and can be linked to responsible social and personal behavior.	More than one objective is written in the affective domain and can be linked to responsible social and personal behavior.	
Teacher Objectives				
Teacher objectives are stated in terms of expected behavior, and are specific and measurable.	No teacher objectives are identified, or teacher objectives are stated as general changes in teaching behaviors.	Teacher objectives are stated in terms of expected behavior and are specific and measurable. Teacher candidate (TC) makes an attempt to meet teacher objectives.	More than two teacher objectives are identified for the lesson and are stated in terms of expected behaviors. Objectives are specific and measurable. TC achieves teacher objectives.	
Plans are identified for adapting and accommodating high- and low-performing students or students with special needs, and the plan is implemented. (NASPE 3.5)	No adaptations or accommodations are planned for or implemented in the lesson. The approach taken is one size fits all, with no differentiation in instruction or practice conditions. No plan is developed for including students with special needs.	Adaptations and accommodations are planned and implemented. Both low- and high-performing students are given various options within the class, such as varying starting/ending points, equipment or grouping. Plans are implemented for students with special needs that allow for effective mainstreaming.	Adaptations and accommodations are planned and implemented. Both low- and high-performing students are given numerous options within the class to extend or refine skills, change equipment or groupings. Plans for students with special needs are implemented and are aligned with student IEPs.	

Instructional Plan	Unacceptable (1 point)	Acceptable (2 points)	Target (3 points)	Score
The learning environment is both physically and psychologically safe. (NASPE 3.5)	Students are singled out during the lesson or placed in situations that could lead to personal embarrassment. TC tolerates inappropriate behavior or allows psychological bullying to occur. Space is not checked for possible safety hazards.	All students are encouraged during the class through positive feedback and constructive criticism. Students participate without being singled out. TC monitors class to eliminate any opportunity for bullying. Space is checked for safety hazards before class begins.	All students are actively engaged in the lesson, with no opportunity for personal embarrassment. TC actively monitors class to encourage students to be supportive of one another. Any possible safety hazards are anticipated and eliminated.	
Learning/practice tasks are progressive and sequential, with refinements, extensions, modification and applications. (NASPE 3.6)	TC plan and implementation includes gaps in progressions. (Steps either are too small or large.) Plan includes only an informing task, and students move immediately into game play without refinements or extensions. Practice tasks are out of sequence.	TC plan and implementation is progressive and sequential, without gaps in progressions. Steps are neither too large nor too small. Informing tasks are followed with refining tasks and extensions. Students move from a series of practice tasks into modified game play before full-sided games.	TC plan and implementation is progressive and sequential, without gaps in progressions. Informing tasks are followed with multiple refining or extensions. TC plans and implements innovative modified games to allow students to practice skills in a game-like environment.	

Instructional Plan	Unacceptable (1 point)	Acceptable (2 points)	Target (3 points)	Score
Lesson has an identifiable opening and closing, and all learning/practice tasks are linked directly to objectives. (NASPE 3.3)	TC does not plan or implement an opening/closing activity. Opening/closing is unrelated to lesson objectives. Multiple tasks in lesson cannot be linked to lesson objectives. Opening or closing does not include checks for understanding, previews or reviews of key components of the lesson. Closing does not allow students to debrief after the lesson.	TC has an identifiable opening/ closing linked to lesson objectives. All tasks in the lesson are linked directly to lesson objectives and provide opportunities for students to achieve objectives of the lesson. Opening and closing include one of the following: preview, review or checks for understanding. Closing allows students the opportunity to debrief after the lesson.	TC has an identifiable opening/ closing linked to lesson objectives. Learning/practice tasks can be linked directly to lesson objectives. TC has at least one application task in the lesson that allows students to integrate various skills/concepts into a modified activity. Opening and closing include two of the following: preview, review or checks for understanding. Students debrief after the lesson.	

Instructional Plan	Unacceptable (1 point)	Acceptable (2 points)	Target (3 points)	Score
Learning/practice tasks provide active, fair and equitable learning environment. (NASPE 3.4)	TC demonstrates behaviors that favor low- or high-performing students (e.g., providing feedback only to skilled performers, allowing low-skilled students to take roles such as scorekeeper or official). Students are not given an equal number of learning/practice opportunities or opportunities to participate in game play. Number of students participating in game or practice opportunities is so large that individual opportunities to participate are limited. Groups of students are disadvantaged in terms of active participation based on gender, class or ethnicity.	TC demonstrates behaviors that create an inclusive environment in which all students are encouraged to participate at their skill levels. Students receive an equal number of learning/practice opportunities. Students receive equal opportunities to receive feedback. TC uses small-sided games and modified practice opportunities to ensure fair and equitable learning experiences for all students.	TC provides opportunities for students to participate in learning/practice tasks based on individual differences and skill levels. Learning/practice tasks are designed to allow various levels of competency to practice at the same time (slanted-rope approach). TC uses multiple types of modified games and activity to ensure active participation for all students. TC accounts for individual differences in planning and implementing the lesson by providing various practice and equipment modifications.	

Instructional Plan	Unacceptable (1 point)	Acceptable (2 points)	Target (3 points)	Score
Teaching plan includes students' use of technology, if appropriate, for lesson objectives. At least one lesson in the unit must include technology. (NASPE 3.7)	No lessons in the unit provide students the opportunity to use technology to enhance their learning/ practice experience. TC makes no use of technology in the unit or in individual lessons.	At least one lesson in the unit has students use technology to enhance the learning/practice task. TC occasionally uses technology during informing tasks.	Two or more lessons in the unit have students use technology to enhance the learning/ practice task. TC consistently uses technology during informing tasks.	
Teaching plan includes demonstrations, skill cues and prompts. (NASPE 4.2)	TC fails to include demonstrations, skill cues or prompts in the plan or in the lesson. TC includes inappropriate skill cues and prompts. (Language or terminology is developmentally inappropriate.) Skill cues or prompts are incorrect for the skill being taught, or demonstration is incorrect.	TC plans and implements demonstrations as part of informing tasks. Lesson plans include developmentally appropriate skill cues and prompts. Skill cues and prompts used during the lesson identify key components of the skill/ concept. Demonstrations are correct.	TC plans and implements demonstrations throughout the lesson and allows students to view demonstration from multiple angles. Skills cues and prompts are developmentally appropriate and well-timed, and identify key components of the skill/concept being taught. TC consistently uses the identified skill cues/ prompts during the lesson.	

Transition/ Management	Unacceptable (1 point)	Acceptable (2 points)	Target (3 points)	Score
Transitions are well-defined in the written plan and are implemented effectively during the lesson. (NASPE 4.5)	TC fails to plan for transitions during the lesson. The length of transitions detracts from academic learning time.	TC plans and implements transitions that take less than 30 seconds. All transitions during the lesson are planned for and executed effectively. TC attempts to reduce the number of transitions needed by sequencing the lesson carefully.	TC plans and implements transitions that consistently take less than 15 seconds. All transitions are planned for and executed using a variety of techniques. TC effectively reduces the number of transitions required in the lesson by planning and sequencing carefully.	
Rules and routines are established and executed effectively. (NASPE 4.5)	TC fails to establish or post developmentally appropriate rules for the classroom. TC has too few or too many rules. TC fails to plan for classroom routines, including the taking of roll, water and bathroom breaks, or equipment collection/distribution. Lack of planning decreases academic learning time.	TC establishes, posts and enforces developmentally appropriate rules for the classroom. TC has established routines for the classroom, including the taking of roll, water and bathroom breaks, and equipment collection/distribution.	TC establishes, posts and consistently enforces developmentally appropriate rules for the classroom. Routines are established and executed for the taking of roll, water and bathroom breaks, and equipment collection/distribution. Careful planning of routines increases academic learning time.	

Assessment	Unacceptable (1 point)	Acceptable (2 points)	Target (3 points)	Score
Assessments are aligned with and appropriate for lesson objectives, and occur throughout the lesson. (NASPE 5.1 & 5.2)	No assessment (either formal or informal) is planned for or used in the lesson. Lesson does not include checks for understanding. Assessments are not aligned with objectives, or are inappropriate measures of objectives. There is a mismatch between the assessment and lesson objectives.	Lesson includes at least two informal assessments and checks for understanding. At least two lessons in the unit include formal assessments, from which data are collected. Assessment occurs at the end of each informing task. Assessments are aligned directly or indirectly with objectives and are appropriate measures of objectives.	Lessons include multiple informal assessments, including checks for understanding. Assessment occurs throughout the lesson. Assessments are aligned directly with objectives and are appropriate measures of objectives.	
Safety/Resources				
Safety is planned for, and strategies are used to ensure students' safety. (NASPE 4.5)	TC fails to check area for potential safety hazards. TC fails to anticipate potential safety issues or provide proactive strategies to ensure students' safety.	TC checks space for potential safety hazards and anticipates potential safety issues. TC identifies proactive strategies to ensure students' physical and psychological safety.	TC checks space for safety hazards and anticipates potential safety issues. TC uses proactive strategies to ensure students' physical and psychological safety.	
Resources used in the lesson are identified using APA format.	TC fails to completely identify source of lesson ideas. Incorrect APA format is used on citation.	TC provides complete information of resources used in lesson by using APA correctly.		

ATTACHMENT 3c
DATA CHART FOR LESSON PLANS, 2008-2009

Undergraduate

SECTION OF THE LESSON PLAN	Application Spring 2009 N = 4			Application Fall 2008 N = 5		
Contextual Factors	UA	AC	TAR	UA	AC	TAR
Lesson Objectives (a): Objectives are performance-based and measurable, and contain three of the four components (action verb, content, criteria or conditions). NASPE/NCATE 3.2		25% 1/4	75% 3/4		60% 3/5	40% 2/5
Lesson Objectives (b): Objectives are developmentally appropriate for the grade/age level. NASPE/NCATE 3.2		25% 1/4	75% 3/4			100% 5/5
Lesson Objectives (c): Objectives are congruent with unit, state and nationals standards. NASPE/NCATE 3.2			100% 4/4		20% 1/5	80% 4/5
Lesson Objectives (d): Lesson has multiple objectives, with at least one objective in each domain of learning.		75% 3/4	25% 1/4		60% 3/5	40% 2/5
Lesson Objectives (e): At least one objective in the affective domain is linked to students' developing responsible social and personal behaviors. NASPE/NCATE 4.6	25% 1/4	75% 3/4			80% 4/5	20% 1/5
Teacher Objectives: Teacher objectives are stated in terms of expected behavior, and are specific and measurable.		25% 1/4	75% 3/4		20% 1/5	80% 4/5
Instructional Plan (a): Plans are identified for adapting and accommodating high- and low-performing students or students with special needs, and the plans are implemented. NASPE/NCATE 3.5	25% 1/4	75% 3/4			60% 3/5	40% 2/5
Instructional Plan (b): Learning environment is both physically and psychologically safe. NASPE/NCATE 3.5		50% 2/4	50% 2/4		20% 1/5	80% 4/5

Undergraduate	Application Spring 2009 N = 4			Application Fall 2008 N = 5		
	UA	AC	TAR	UA	AC	TAR
SECTION OF THE LESSON PLAN						
Instructional Plan (c): Learning/practice tasks are progressive and sequential, with refinements, extensions, modification and applications. NASPE/NCATE 3.6		50% 2/4	50% 2/4		80% 4/5	20% 1/5
Instructional Plan (d): Lesson has an identifiable opening/closing, and all learning/practice tasks are linked directly to objectives. NASPE/NCATE 3.3		50% 2/4	50% 2/4			100% 5/5
Instructional Plan (e): Learning/practice tasks provide an active, fair and equitable learning environment. NASPE/NCATE 3.4		75% 3/4	25% 1/4		20% 1/5	80% 4/5
Instructional Plan (f): Teaching plan includes students' use of technology, if appropriate, for lesson objectives. NASPE/NCATE 3.7		50% 2/4	50% 2/4		80% 4/5	20% 1/5
Instructional Plan (g): Teaching plan includes demonstrations, skill cues and prompts. NASPE/NCATE 4.2		50% 2/4	50% 2/4		20% 1/5	80% 4/5
Transition/Management (a): Transitions are well-defined in the written plan and are implemented effectively during the lesson. NASPE/NCATE 4.5		25% 1/4	75% 3/4		60% 3/5	40% 2/5
Transition/Management (b): Rules and routines are established and executed effectively. NASPE/NCATE 4.5		75% 3/4	25% 1/4		20% 1/5	80% 4/5
Assessment: Assessments are aligned with and appropriate for lesson objectives, and occur throughout the lesson. NASPE/NCATE 5.1 & 5.2		75% 3/4	25% 1/4		60% 3/5	40% 2/5
Safety: Safety is planned for and strategies are used to ensure students' safety. NASPE/NCATE 4.5		50% 2/4	50% 2/4			100% 5/5
Resources: Resources used in the lesson are identified using APA format.		50% 2/4	50% 2/4		20% 1/5	80% 4/5

Each candidate is evaluated on five separate lessons plans that were implemented. The final designation of level is determined by the range listed below for the mean of the five lesson plans during each experience. Only lesson plans that are implemented are evaluated for inclusion in this data chart. 3.00 – 2.50 = Target (Average on 5 lesson plans with 3 = target, 2 = acceptable, and 1 = unacceptable on each item on the rubric); 2.49 – 2.0 = Acceptable; 1.99 and below = Unacceptable. *Candidates must score in the acceptable range on all components of the lesson plan rubric during their internship.

Appendix E

Teacher Candidate Artifact Approval Form Template

Teacher Candidate:

Submission of Assessment/Assignment Date:

Assessment/Assignment:

Evaluator:

I give permission for this assessment/assignment to be used by the department as a teacher candidate artifact for purposes such as serving as an exemplar, for program review, for program accreditation and/or for departmental annual review reports.

Signature   Date

Appendix F

Alignment of Standards & Courses Matrix

NASPE Initial PETE Standards and Elements (2008)

Appendix F

ALIGNMENT OF STANDARDS & COURSES MATRIX
NASPE Initial PETE Standards and Elements (2008)

Standard/Elements	Courses
P = Primary focus S = Secondary focus C = Cursory focus	
Standard 1: Scientific and Theoretical Knowledge Physical education teacher candidates know and apply discipline-specific scientific and theoretical concepts critical to the development of physically educated individuals.	
Element 1.1 Describe and apply physiological and biomechanical concepts related to skillful movement, physical activity and fitness.	
Element 1.2 Describe and apply motor learning and psychological/behavioral theory related to skillful movement, physical activity and fitness.	
Element 1.3 Describe and apply motor development theory and principles related to skillful movement, physical activity and fitness.	
Element 1.4 Identify historical, philosophical and social perspectives of physical education issues and legislation.	
Element 1.5 Analyze and correct critical elements of motor skills and performance concepts.	
Standard 2: Skill-Based and Fitness-Based Competence Physical education teacher candidates are physically educated individuals with the knowledge and skills necessary to demonstrate competent movement performance and health-enhancing fitness as delineated in the NASPE K-12 Standards.	
Element 2.1 Demonstrate personal competence in motor skill performance for a variety of physical activities and movement patterns.	
Element 2.2 Achieve and maintain a health-enhancing level of fitness throughout the program.	
Element 2.3 Demonstrate performance concepts related to skillful movement in a variety of physical activities.	

Standard/Elements	Courses														
P = Primary focus S = Secondary focus C = Cursory focus															
Standard 3: Planning and Implementation Physical education teacher candidates plan and implement developmentally appropriate learning experiences aligned with local, state and national standards to address the diverse needs of all students.															
Element 3.1 Design and implement short- and long-term plans that are linked to program and instructional goals, as well as a variety of student needs.															
Element 3.2 Develop and implement appropriate (e.g., measurable, developmentally appropriate, performance-based) goals and objectives aligned with local, state and/or national standards.															
Element 3.3 Design and implement content that is aligned with lesson objectives.															
Element 3.4 Plan for and manage resources to provide active, fair and equitable learning experiences.															
Element 3.5 Plan and adapt instruction for diverse student needs, adding specific accommodations and/or modifications for student exceptionalities.															
Element 3.6 Plan and implement progressive and sequential instruction that addresses the diverse needs of all students.															
Element 3.7 Demonstrate knowledge of current technology by planning and implementing learning experiences that require students to appropriately use technology to meet lesson objectives.															

P = Primary focus
S = Secondary focus
C = Cursory focus

Standard/Elements	Courses
Standard 4: Instructional Delivery and Management Physical education teacher candidates use effective communication and pedagogical skills and strategies to enhance student engagement and learning.	
Element 4.1 Demonstrate effective verbal and non-verbal communication skills across a variety of instructional formats.	
Element 4.2 Implement effective demonstrations, explanations and instructional cues and prompts to link physical activity concepts to appropriate learning experiences.	
Element 4.3 Provide effective instructional feedback for skill acquisition, student learning and motivation.	
Element 4.4 Recognize the changing dynamics of the environment and adjust instructional tasks based on student responses.	
Element 4.5 Use managerial rules, routines and transitions to create and maintain a safe and effective learning environment.	
Element 4.6 Implement strategies to help students demonstrate responsible personal and social behaviors in a productive learning environment.	
Standard 5: Impact on Student Learning Physical education teacher candidates use assessments and reflection to foster student learning and inform instructional decisions.	
Element 5.1 Select or create appropriate assessments that will measure student achievement of goals and objectives.	
Element 5.2 Use appropriate assessments to evaluate student learning before, during and after instruction.	
Element 5.3 Use the reflective cycle to implement change in teacher performance, student learning and/or instructional goals and decisions.	

Standard/Elements	Courses														
P = Primary focus S = Secondary focus C = Cursory focus															
Standard 6: Professionalism Physical education teacher candidates demonstrate dispositions essential to becoming effective professionals.															
Element 6.1 Demonstrate behaviors that are consistent with the belief that all students can become physically educated individuals.															
Element 6.2 Participate in activities that enhance collaboration and lead to professional growth and development.															
Element 6.3 Demonstrate behaviors that are consistent with the professional ethics of highly qualified teachers.															
Element 6.4 Communicate in ways that convey respect and sensitivity.															

Appendix G

Standards/Course Assessment Matrix

NASPE Initial PETE Standards and Elements (2008)

Appendix G

STANDARDS/COURSE ASSESSMENT MATRIX
NASPE Initial PETE Standards and Elements (2008)

Standard/Elements	Assessments
P = Primary focus S = Secondary focus C = Cursory focus	- Courses in which primary focus is indicated, or a secondary focus if no primary focus is indicated - Provide a **minimum of at least 3 assessments** per standard - Use the following format: Course number: Name of Assessment [specific element/ number addressed; e.g., 1.2]
Standard 1: Scientific and Theoretical Knowledge Physical education teacher candidates know and apply discipline-specific scientific and theoretical concepts critical to the development of physically educated individuals.	
Element 1.1 Describe and apply physiological and biomechanical concepts related to skillful movement, physical activity and fitness.	
Element 1.2 Describe and apply motor learning and psychological/ behavioral theory related to skillful movement, physical activity and fitness.	
Element 1.3 Describe and apply motor development theory and principles related to skillful movement, physical activity and fitness.	
Element 1.4 Identify historical, philosophical and social perspectives of physical education issues and legislation.	
Element 1.5 Analyze and correct critical elements of motor skills and performance concepts.	

Standard/Elements	Assessments
P = Primary focus S = Secondary focus C = Cursory focus	- Courses in which primary focus is indicated, or a secondary focus if no primary focus is indicated - Provide a **minimum of at least 3 assessments** per standard - Use the following format: Course number: Name of Assessment [specific element/ number addressed; e.g., 1.2]
Standard 2: Skill-Based and Fitness-Based Competence Physical education teacher candidates are physically educated individuals with the knowledge and skills necessary to demonstrate competent movement performance and health-enhancing fitness as delineated in the NASPE K-12 Standards.	
Element 2.1 Demonstrate personal competence in motor skill performance for a variety of physical activities and movement patterns.	
Element 2.2 Achieve and maintain a health-enhancing level of fitness throughout the program.	
Element 2.3 Demonstrate performance concepts related to skillful movement in a variety of physical activities.	

Standard 2 Note: *Without discrimination against those with disabilities, physical education teacher candidates with special needs are allowed and encouraged to use a variety of accommodations and/or modifications to demonstrate competent movement and performance concepts (e.g., modified/adapted equipment, augmented communication devices, multi-media devices) and fitness (e.g., weight training programs, exercise logs).

Standard/Elements	Assessments
P = Primary focus S = Secondary focus C = Cursory focus	- Courses in which primary focus is indicated, or a secondary focus if no primary focus is indicated - Provide a **minimum of at least 3 assessments** per standard - Use the following format: 　Course number: Name of Assessment [specific outcome/element/indicator number addressed]
Standard 3: Planning and Implementation Physical education teacher candidates plan and implement developmentally appropriate learning experiences aligned with local, state and national standards to address the diverse needs of all students.	
Element 3.1 Design and implement short- and long-term plans that are linked to program and instructional goals, as well as a variety of student needs.	
Element 3.2 Develop and implement appropriate (e.g., measurable, developmentally appropriate, performance-based) goals and objectives aligned with local, state and/or national standards.	
Element 3.3 Design and implement content that is aligned with lesson objectives.	
Element 3.4 Plan for and manage resources to provide active, fair and equitable learning experiences.	
Element 3.5 Plan and adapt instruction for diverse student needs, adding specific accommodations and/or modifications for student exceptionalities.	
Element 3.6 Plan and implement progressive and sequential instruction that addresses the diverse needs of all students.	
Element 3.7 Demonstrate knowledge of current technology by planning and implementing learning experiences that require students to appropriately use technology to meet lesson objectives.	

Standard/Elements	Assessments
P = Primary focus S = Secondary focus C = Cursory focus	- Courses in which primary focus is indicated, or a secondary focus if no primary focus is indicated - Provide a **minimum of at least 3 assessments** per standard - Use the following format: Course number: Name of Assessment [specific outcome/element/indicator number addressed]
Standard 4: Instructional Delivery and Management Physical education teacher candidates use effective communication and pedagogical skills and strategies to enhance student engagement and learning.	
Element 4.1 Demonstrate effective verbal and non-verbal communication skills across a variety of instructional formats.	
Element 4.2 Implement effective demonstrations, explanations and instructional cues and prompts to link physical activity concepts to appropriate learning experiences.	
Element 4.3 Provide effective instructional feedback for skill acquisition, student learning and motivation.	
Element 4.4 Recognize the changing dynamics of the environment and adjust instructional tasks based on student responses.	
Element 4.5 Use managerial rules, routines and transitions to create and maintain a safe and effective learning environment.	
Element 4.6 Implement strategies to help students demonstrate responsible personal and social behaviors in a productive learning environment.	
Standard 5: Impact on Student Learning Physical education teacher candidates use assessments and reflection to foster student learning and inform instructional decisions.	
Element 5.1 Select or create appropriate assessments that will measure student achievement of goals and objectives.	
Element 5.2 Use appropriate assessments to evaluate student learning before, during and after instruction.	
Element 5.3 Use the reflective cycle to implement change in teacher performance, student learning and/or instructional goals and decisions.	

Standard/Elements	Assessments
P = Primary focus S = Secondary focus C = Cursory focus	- Courses in which primary focus is indicated, or a secondary focus if no primary focus is indicated - Provide a **minimum of at least 3 assessments** per standard - Use the following format: Course number: Name of Assessment [specific outcome/element/indicator number addressed]
Standard 6: Professionalism Physical education teacher candidates demonstrate dispositions that are essential to becoming effective professionals.	
Element 6.1 Demonstrate behaviors that are consistent with the belief that all students can become physically educated individuals.	
Element 6.2 Participate in activities that enhance collaboration and lead to professional growth and development.	
Element 6.3 Demonstrate behaviors that are consistent with the professional ethics of highly qualified teachers.	
Element 6.4 Communicate in ways that convey respect and sensitivity.	

*The term "teacher candidate" refers to pre-service teachers in an initial preparation program. The term "students" refers to P-12 students.